ECG for the Small Animal Practitioner

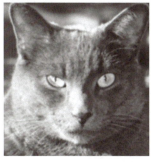

Editor: Carroll C. Cann

Managing Editor: Cynthia J. Roantree

Design: Finegan/Thompson Design

Teton NewMedia

P.O. Box 4833

Jackson, Wyoming 83001

1-888-770-3165

www.tetonnm.com

PRINTED IN THE UNITED STATES OF AMERICA

ISBN 1-893441-00-8

Print number 5

Dedication

To my wife Jeri, and my son Kyle,

and to all my students of electrocardiography

for whom this book is written.

Larry Patrick Tilley

To my mother Beryl,

who continues to nurture my independent

spirit and deep love of learning,

and to my brother David,

who shares my delight in figuring out

how things work.

Naomi Lee Burtnick

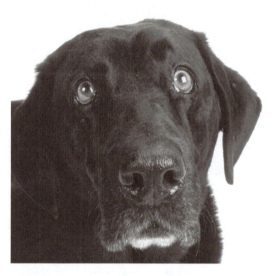

VetMed
Dr. Larry P. Tilley & Associates
Suite 279
1704-B Llano Street
Santa Fe, New Mexico, 87505   USA
Telephone: 505-424-9731
Fax: 505-424-8752
Email: tilleyvetmed@earthlink.net

Within the United States:
Telephone: 800-214-9760
Fax: 800-820-6815

Preface

We take great satisfaction

in bringing the reader this convenient review of basic canine and feline electrocardiography. It is our hope that the text will both help the practicing veterinarian meet his day-to-day needs and stimulate the interest of students in small animal electrocardiography. We feel that the conciseness and clarity of this presentation has contributed immeasurably to these ends.

We also want to acknowledge thanks to Williams and Wilkins for permission to reuse selected illustrations from my Textbook: *Essentials of Canine and Feline Electrocardiography, Interpretation and Treatment*, 3rd Edition, Lea & Febiger, 1992.

The rapid evolution of animal electrocardiography has made an easily accessible text such as this both necessary and welcome. Today's ECG instruments have placed in the hands of the veterinarian an accurate and efficient means of recording the electrical activity of the animal's heart. But what does the ECG tracing mean? To own an electrocardiograph is not enough; the veterinarian must use his ECG instrument correctly and interpret the ECG recording accurately.

Table of Contents

Section 1 "How To"

Section 2 -Electrocardiographic Examples

Normal Sinus Impulse Formation

Disturbances of Sinus Impulse Formation

Disturbances of Supraventricular Impulse Formation

Disturbances of Ventricular Impulse Formation

Disturbances of Impulse Conduction

Escape Rhythms

Miscellaneous Disturbances

Appendix

Section 1
"How To"

Introduction

The goal of this book

is to provide you with fundamental information and interpretation techniques that will help you differentiate between normal, abnormal, and life-threatening electrocardiographic arrhythmias in the dog and cat.

Even with the advent of newer technology for assessing cardiac function, such as echocardiography, the electrocardiogram remains the definitive tool for diagnosing arrhythmias. It is to that end that we have focused this book. By carefully following the simplified techniques outlined here, you will easily build the foundation for recognizing and treating most arrhythmias.

Some Helpful Hints

Scattered throughout the text you will find the following symbols to help you focus on what is really important.

✓ This is a routine feature of the subject being discussed. We've tried to narrow it down, honest.

♥ This is a salient feature. If you remember anything about this particular subject, this is it.

🔑 We'll use this selectively. It's a key to understanding the whole process of ECG interpretation.

✋ Stop. This doesn't look important but it can really make a difference when trying to sort out unusual situations.

💣 Something serious, possibly life-threatening will happen if you don't remember this. For example, this book could blow up.

Applications of the Electrocardiogram

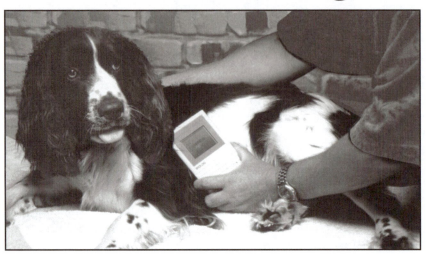

♥ Exact diagnoses of arrhythmias heard on auscultation.

✓ Acute onset of dyspnea.

✓ Shock.

✓ Fainting or seizures.

✓ Monitoring during and after surgery (for depth of anesthesia as well as cardiac monitoring).

✓ All cardiac murmurs.

✓ Cardiomegaly found on thoracic radiographs.

✓ Cyanosis.

✓ Preoperatively in older animals.

✓ Evaluating the effect of cardiac drugs–especially digitalis, quinidine, and propranolol.

✓ Electrolyte disturbances, especially potassium abnormalities.

✓ Periocardiocentesis, for monitoring purposes.

✓ Systemic diseases that affect the heart (e.g., pyometra, pancreatitis, uremia, neoplasia), with toxic myocarditis and resulting arrhythmias.

✓ Basis for records and consultation.

✓ Serial ECGs as an aid in the prognosis and diagnosis of cardiac disease.

Circulation System

✓ The body depends on the heart pumping oxygenated blood to the tissues.

✓ Unoxygenated blood enters the right side of the heart and is pumped to the lungs (pulmonary circulation).

✓ From the lungs, the newly oxygenated blood enters the left side of the heart where it is pumped to the organs and tissues via the systemic circulation.

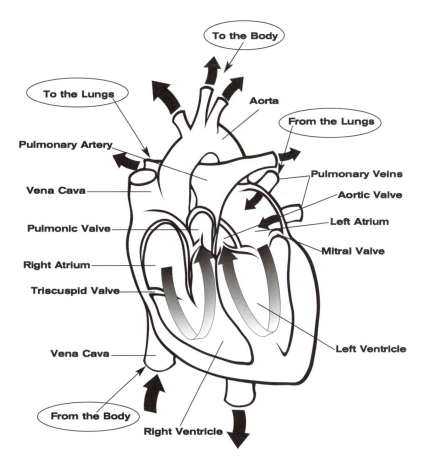

Conduction System

Electrical impulses are transmitted through the heart via specialized conduction cells in the following sequence:

✓ Sinoatrial node.

✓ Interatrial and internodal conduction tracts.

✓ Atrioventricular (AV) node.

✓ Bundle of His (the region of the AV node and the Bundle of His is called the AV junction).

✓ The left and right bundle branches.

✓ Purkinje fibers.

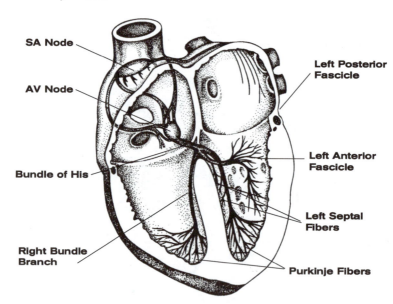

What is depolarization and repolarization?

Depolarization–heart muscle contraction in response to electrical stimulus. Occurs when electrolytes move across the cell membrane (sodium/potassium pump).

Repolarization–heart muscle relaxation occurs when the electrolytes move back across the cell membrane rendering the cell ready for the next electrical impulse.

Five Physiologic Properties of Cardiac Muscle

Automaticity

Sinoatrial node is the primary pacemaker of the heart, but any cells of the conduction system can initiate their own impulses under the right circumstances.

♥ As a rule, the further down in the conduction system the slower the rate of automaticity.

Excitability

✓ Cardiac muscle is excited when the electrical stimulus reduces the resting potential to the threshold potential.

✓ The degree of the resting potential within the cell determines its excitability and obeys the "all-or-none" law.

Refractoriness

✓ Heart muscle will not respond to external stimuli during its period of contraction.

Conductivity

✓ Activation of an individual muscle cell produces activity in the neighboring muscle cell.

✓ Conduction velocity varies in the different portions of the specialized conduction system and muscle fibers.

♥ Velocity is greatest in the Purkinje fibers and least in the mid-portion of the AV node.

✓ Activation sequence is so arranged that the maximum mechanical efficiency is provided from each corresponding contraction.

Contractility

✓ Occurs in response to electrical current.

♥ Remember that the ECG only measures the stimulus for contraction–not the actual contraction itself. Echocardiography is the tool of choice for assessing contractility.

Electrocardiogram

Definition–Graphic recording of electrical potentials produced by heart muscle during the different phases of the cardiac cycle.

✓ The voltage variations are produced by depolarization and repolarization of individual muscle cells.

✓ Each portion of the electrocardiogram thus arises from a specific anatomic or physiologic area of the heart.

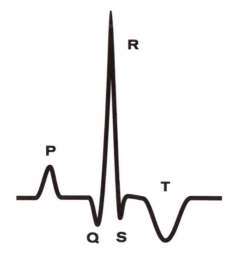

P wave–corresponds to atrial depolarization or contraction.
   P waves can be positive, negative, or biphasic depending on the lead (we'll explain leads just a little later).

QRS waves–correspond to ventricular depolarization or contraction.
   Q wave is the first negative deflection.

   R wave is the first positive deflection.

   S wave is the negative deflection that follows the R wave.

T wave–represents ventricular repolarization or relaxation.
   T waves can be positive, negative or biphasic.
   ✋ Every QRS complex *has* to have a T wave following it.

What is a Lead, anyway?

✓ Lead systems allow you to look at the heart from different angles. Each different angle is called a lead. The different leads can be compared to radiographs taken from different angles, such as lateral and dorsoventral thoracic radiographs taken for evaluation of cardiac chambers.

♥ Each lead has a positive and negative pole attached to the surface of the skin, which can then be used to measure the spread of electrical activity within the heart.

Upward deflection on the ECG–is produced when electrical impulses travel towards a positive electrode.

Downward deflection on the ECG–is produced when electrical impulses travel towards a negative electrode.

Flat line (isoelectric line)–is produced when there is no electrical spread through the heart, or if the electrical forces are equal.

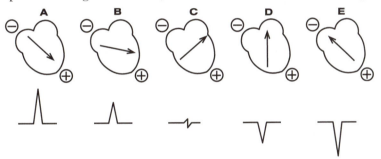

✓ To determine the mean electrical axis (useful in assessing cardiac chamber size) it is necessary to run the 3 standard bipolar leads as well as the 3 augmented unipolar limb leads.

Lead I–right arm (-) compared to left arm (+)

Lead II–right arm (-) compared to left leg (+)

Lead III–left arm (-) compared to left leg (+)

aVR–right arm (+) compared to a point halfway between left arm and left leg (-)

aVL–left arm (+) compared to a point halfway between right arm and left leg (-)

aVF–left leg (+) compared to a point halfway between left arm and right arm (-)

♥ The good news is that we only need to use lead II to assess arrhythmias.

Generation of the Electrocardiogram

The following illustrations depict the genesis of the ECG on the basis of:

✓ Initiation of the impulse in the primary pacemaker (sinoatrial node).

✓ Transmission of the impulse through the specialized conduction system of the heart.

✓ Activation or depolarization of the atrial and ventricular myocardium.

✓ Recovery or repolarization of the preceding three areas.

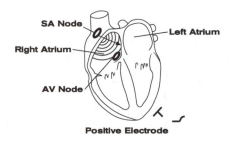

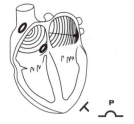

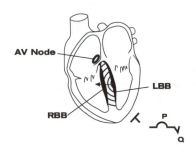

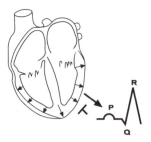

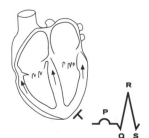

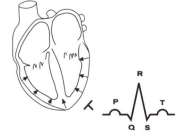

Electrocardiographic Recording Technique

Patient cable–a single lead or 6-lead patient cable can be attached to a hand-held recorder/monitor or any standard ECG strip chart recorder, and the ECG can be recorded with the patient in lateral or standing position. The electrode clips are attached directly to the skin and moistened with alcohol or gel to assure good contact.

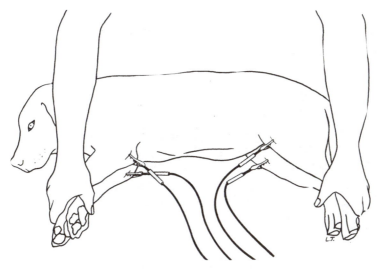

✓ Record lead II for 30-60 seconds at 25 mm/sec to assess arrhythmias

✓ Record a brief tracing at 50 mm/sec for ease of measurement of P-QRS-T waveforms.

✓ While the ECG is recording the following should be observed:

  1. Center the recording on the paper so that both the top and bottom of the waveforms can be seen. Adjust the position control if the tracing wanders.

  2. Decrease the sensitivity to ½ cm = 1 mv if the QRS complexes go off the paper.

  3. Increase the length of the tracing if an arrhythmia is seen.

  4. R waves should be positive on lead I. If negative, check the lead wires to determine whether they are attached to the correct limbs. If connections are correct, then a true abnormality exists.

17

Electrocardiographic Recording Technique (continued)

Direct chest placement–a hand-held ECG recorder/monitor allows direct chest placement.

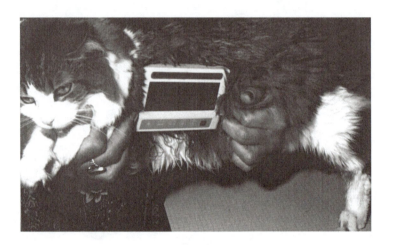

✓ Wet the animal's coat with alcohol or place gel on the electrode plates, and then position the unit on the chest.

✓ The tracing is seen on the monitor and stored for printing later with one of the following options:

1. Strip printer.

2. Printer interface to a standard inkjet printer for a plain paper printout.

3. Direct download to PC computer program.

ECG Paper & Standardization

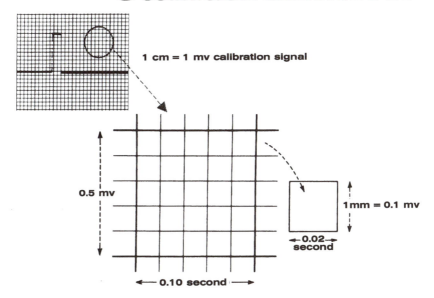

1 cm = 1 mv calibration signal

0.5 mv

1mm = 0.1 mv

0.02 second

0.10 second

Standardization Signal

✓ Without a standardization signal, the ECG paper is merely graph paper. By entering a signal, you place value on each of the smallest squares.

✋ At 1 cm = 1 mv each tiny square represents 0.1 mv in height (amplitude) and 0.02 seconds in width (duration) at a paper speed of 50 mm/sec. It wouldn't be such a bad idea to memorize this.

✓ The calibration signal can be changed, if necessary, to affect the amplitude only. If the complexes are very tall and extend beyond the margins of the paper, the signal can be reduced to 0.5 cm = 1 mv. With very small amplitude complexes, the standardization can be increased to 2 cm = 1 mv and the height of the complexes will increase accordingly.

Time markings–ECG paper also has time markings in the margin every 1.5 sec at 50 mm/sec. An example of the time markings is shown in the section on calculating heart rate.

All ECGs in this book will be at a paper speed of 50 mm/sec and at a calibration of 1 cm = 1 mv.

Calculating the Heart Rate

The heart rate (beats/minute) can be calculated easily by:

1. Using the ECG ruler on the next page. The ruler allows you to use 25 mm/sec or 50 mm/sec paper speed.

2. Or, by counting the number of beats (R-R intervals) between two sets of marks in the margin of the ECG paper (3 seconds at 50 mm/sec) and multiplying by 20.

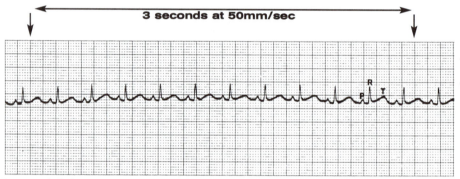

3 seconds at 50mm/sec

Normal feline ECG: 11 beats X 20 = 220 beats/minute

Regardless of which system you use it is important to know the correct paper speed!

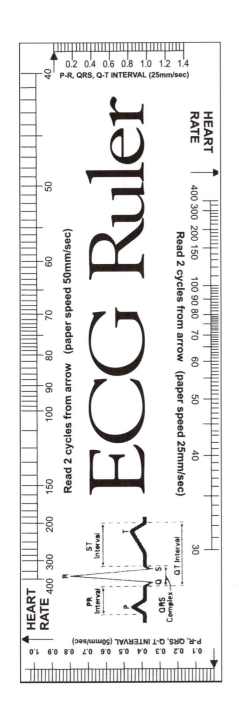

Use the enclosed ruler in the Inside Back Cover for an easy way to measure heart rate & P-QRS-T intervals

Measuring the P-QRS-T

P wave–represents depolarization of the atria, and its duration indicates the time required for an impulse to pass from the sinoatrial (SA) node to the atrioventricular (AV) node.

✓ The normal P wave on lead II is small, positive and rounded.

✓ It is measured from the upper edge of the baseline to the top of the P wave.

✓ The width of the P wave is measured at its inside, from the start to the end of the deflection from the baseline.

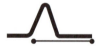

P-R interval–reflects activation of the AV junction.

✓ It is measured from the beginning of the P wave to the beginning of the Q wave (R wave, if no Q wave is present).

QRS complex–represents depolarization of the ventricles.

✓ The width of QRS complex is measured from the beginning of the first deflection to the end of the final deflection of the complex.

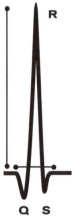

Measuring the P-QRS-T(continued)

✔ The height of the R wave is measured from the top edge of the baseline to the peak of the R wave.

✔ The depth of the Q or S wave is measured from the bottom edge of the baseline to the lowest part of the Q or S, respectively.

S-T segment–represents the time interval from the end of the QRS interval to the onset of the T wave, the early phase of ventricular repolarization.

✔ It may be above, at, or below the level of the baseline.

✔ Only significant elevations or depressions from baseline should be considered abnormal.

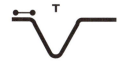

T wave–is the first major deflection following the QRS complex and represents repolarization of the ventricles.

✔ It may be positive, notched, negative, or diphasic.

✔ T wave should be less than 25 % of the QRS amplitude.

Q-T interval–is the summation of ventricular depolarization and repolarization and represents ventricular systole.

✔ Q-T interval is measured from the onset of the Q wave to the end of the T wave.

✔ The Q-T interval alone in veterinary medicine is not often helpful in diagnosis.

Canine ECG Normal Values*

Rate
70 to 160 beats/min for adult dogs
60 to 140 beats/min for giant breeds
Up to 180 beats/min for toy breeds
Up to 220 beats/min for puppies

Rhythm
Normal sinus rhythm/Sinus arrhythmia
Wandering sinus pacemaker

P wave
Width: maximum, 0.04 sec (2 boxes wide)
        maximum, 0.05 sec (2½ boxes wide) in giant breeds
Height: maximum, 0.4 mv (4 boxes tall)

P-R interval
Width: 0.06 to 0.13 sec (3 to 6½ boxes)

QRS complex
Width: maximum, 0.05 sec (2½ boxes) in small breeds
        maximum, 0.06 sec (3 boxes) in large breeds
Height of R wave: maximum, 3.0 mv (30 boxes) in large breeds
        maximum, 2.5 mv (25 boxes) in small breeds

S-T segment
No depression: not more than 0.2 mv (2 boxes)
No elevation: not more than 0.15 mv (1½ boxes)

T wave
Can be positive, negative, or diphasic
Not greater than ¼ amplitude of R wave

Q-T interval
Width: 0.15 to 0.25 sec (7 ½ - 12 ½ boxes) at normal heart rate

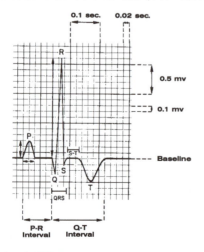

* Lead II:
50 mm/sec,
1 cm = 1 mv

Feline ECG Normal Values*

Rate
    120 to 240 beats/min

Rhythm
    Normal sinus rhythm
    Sinus tachycardia (physiologic reaction to excitement)

P wave
    Width: maximum, 0.04 sec (2 boxes wide)
    Height: maximum, 0.2 mv (2 boxes tall)

P-R interval
    Width: 0.05 to 0.09 sec (2½ to 4½ boxes)

QRS complex
    Width: maximum, 0.04 sec (2 boxes)
    Height of R wave: maximum, 0.9 mv (9 boxes)

S-T segment
    No depression or elevation

T wave
    Can be positive, negative, or diphasic; most often positive
    Maximum amplitude: 0.3 mv (3 boxes)

Q-T interval
    Width: 0.12 to 0.18 sec (6 to 9 boxes) at normal heart rate

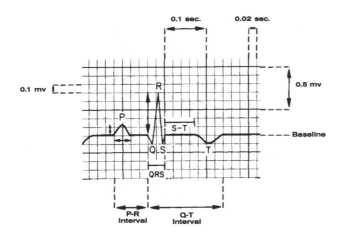

*Lead II: 50 mm/sec, 1 cm = 1 mv

Quick & Dirty Guide to ECG Enlargements & Bundle Branch Blocks

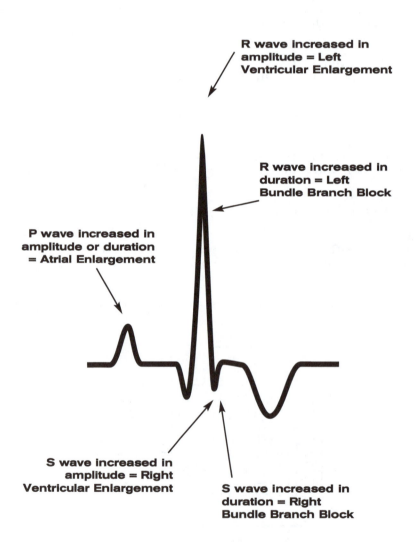

R wave increased in amplitude = Left Ventricular Enlargement

R wave increased in duration = Left Bundle Branch Block

P wave increased in amplitude or duration = Atrial Enlargement

S wave increased in amplitude = Right Ventricular Enlargement

S wave increased in duration = Right Bundle Branch Block

Classification of Arrhythmias

Definition of Arrhythmias:

1. An abnormality in the rate, regularity, or site of origin of the cardiac impulse.
2. A disturbance in conduction of the impulse such that the normal sequence of activation of the atria and ventricles is altered.

Classification of Arrhythmias

Abnormalities of impulse formation or impulse conduction are the basis for the following classification:

Normal sinus impulse formation

Normal sinus rhythm
Sinus arrhythmia

Disturbances of sinus impulse formation

Sinus bradycardia
Sinus tachycardia

Disturbances of supraventricular impulse formation

Atrial premature complexes
Atrial tachycardia
Atrial fibrillation
Atrioventricular junctional premature complexes
Atrioventricular junctional tachycardia

Disturbances of ventricular impulse formation

Ventricular premature complexes
Ventricular tachycardia
Ventricular asystole
Ventricular fibrillation

Disturbances of impulse conduction

Sinus arrest or block
Sick sinus syndrome
Atrial standstill
Ventricular pre-excitation
First-degree atrioventricular block
Second-degree atrioventricular block
Third-degree atrioventricular block
Left bundle branch block
Right bundle branch block

Building Blocks for Arrhythmia Interpretation

There are two basic building blocks for placing an arrhythmia within the classification presented earlier.

✓ Recognizing the site of origin of the abnormal beat.
✓ Recognizing deviations from the normal rate of automaticity for that site.

1. Site of origin

Three different sites can be identified on lead II by the following features:

Atrial–positive deflection P waves are present with a constant P-R interval and a normal duration QRS complex.*

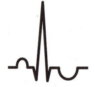

   ✓Ectopic atrial origin beats have all the same features as a normally conducted SA nodal origin beat. The primary difference lies in the timing.

Junctional–negative deflection P waves, or no P waves, with a normally conducted, short-duration QRS complex.*

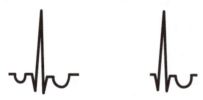

Ventricular–no P waves are evident. QRS complexes are wide and bizarre appearing and may be positive or negative polarity, depending on which ventricle is the site of origin.

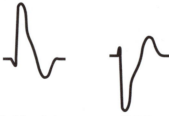

*If a bundle branch block is present, QRS complexes will have prolonged duration and poor morphology.

28

Building Blocks for Arrhythmia
Interpretation (continued)

2. Intrinsic rates of automaticity

Atrial, junctional, and ventricular sites each have a normal rate of automaticity (the ability to initiate impulses), but may respond in the following abnormal ways:

> Too fast (tachycardia)
> Too slow (bradycardia)
> Too irritable (premature)
> Absent (block)

♥ **Normal pacemaker rates in the dog:**

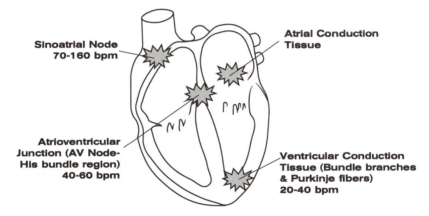

**Sinoatrial Node
70-160 bpm**

**Atrial Conduction
Tissue**

**Atrioventricular
Junction (AV Node-
His bundle region)
40-60 bpm**

**Ventricular Conduction
Tissue (Bundle branches
& Purkinje fibers)
20-40 bpm**

✓ In cats, the SA nodal/atrial intrinsic rate of automaticity is 120-240 bpm, with the normal junctional and ventricular sites having proportionately slower rates.

✓ *Passive arrhythmias (escape rhythms)*—rates slower than the SA node occur because of SA nodal depression, allowing "escapes" of other pacemakers from its influence.

✓ *Active arrhythmias*—occur when a normally functioning SA node is not able to act as the pacemaker because other pacemakers are abnormally forming impulses at a faster rate.

✓ Both passive and active arrhythmias may be intermittent or persistent, repetitive, or occurring in varying combinations.

Rule of thumb: Whichever site is fastest will drive the heart!

Interpreting
Arrhythmias—the Easy Way

Arrhythmias can be intimidating. Therefore, it is important that we find a simple approach for analyzing rhythm strips. Systematically following the five-step method outlined below has proven to be both easy and effective.

Step 1. Calculate the heart rate
✓ Decide whether the heart rate is rapid, slow, or normal. Here's your chance to try that new ECG ruler.

Step 2. Assess the rhythm
✓ Scan the strip from left to right, noting if the R-R intervals are regular or irregular.
✓ A caliper is a handy tool for plotting P-P and R-R intervals.

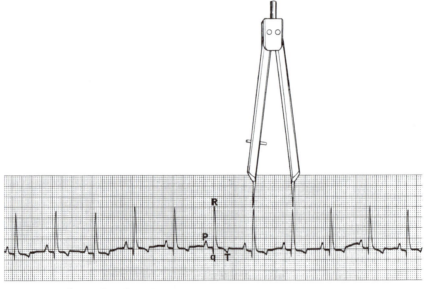

Step 3. Identify the P waves
✓ *Normal P wave (positive and rounded on Lead II)*—indicates that the impulse is originating in the SA node.
✓ *P wave that differs from normal in shape and is upright*—may represent an ectopic pacemaker in the atrium.
✓ *P waves that are inverted*—on lead II, indicate that the impulse was formed in or near the atrioventricular junction.
✓ *Absence of P waves*—signifies atrial fibrillation, atrial standstill, or buried P waves in QRS complexes of AV junctional rhythms.
✓ *P waves can be superimposed*—on a portion of the QRS complex, S-T segment, or T wave of the preceding cardiac cycle in various supraventricular tachycardias.

Interpreting Arrhythmias–
the Easy Way (continued)

Step 4. Assess QRS shape and duration

✓ *Normal duration QRS complexes*–identical to those recorded before an arrhythmia, indicate normal activation of the ventricles. These complexes are either formed in the SA node or from an abnormal site anywhere above the bundle of His.

✓ *Wide QRS complexes*–with various configurations indicate an ectopic pacemaker below the bundle of His (ventricular) or a lesion in the intraventricular conduction system (bundle branch block).

Step 5. Relationship between P waves & QRS complexes

✓ Normally, there should be one P wave for every QRS complex, with a constant P-R interval.

✓ P waves may precede normal QRS complexes by different time spans.

> *Long P-R intervals*–indicate an AV conduction delay (1° AV block).

> *Short P-R intervals*–are seen with accessory conduction around the AV node, or in AV junctional rhythms in which the P wave is positioned close to the QRS complex.

> *P wave not followed by a QRS complex*–an AV block (2° AV block) has occurred. If the P-R interval lengthens gradually until a P wave occurs without a succeeding QRS complex, another form of 2° AV block has occurred.

> *P-R intervals vary*–in 3° AV block the relationship of the atria and ventricles is interrupted. One impulse forming site is the SA node; the other is an independent ventricular escape rhythm.

Last step: Name that arrhythmia

✓ Place the arrhythmia within the classification.

✓ The best name for an arrhythmia always identifies exactly which part of the heart is not working properly.

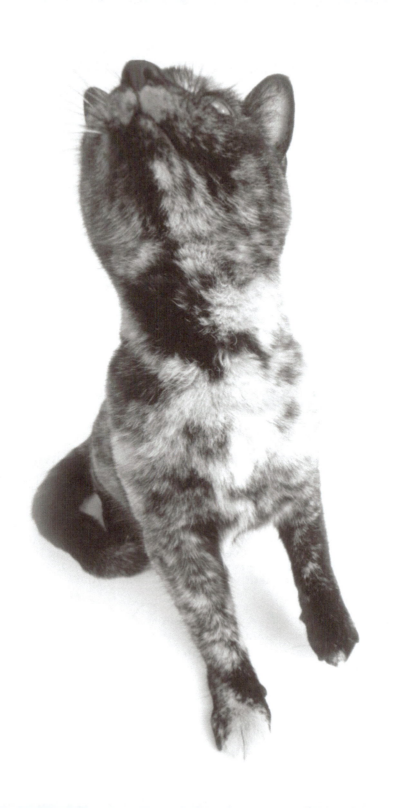

Section 2
Electro-cardiographic Examples

Normal Sinus Impulse Formation

✓ Normal Sinus Rhythm
✓ Sinus Arrhythmia

Disturbances of Sinus Impulse Formation

✓ Sinus Bradycardia
✓ Sinus Tachycardia

Normal Sinus Rhythm

Dog

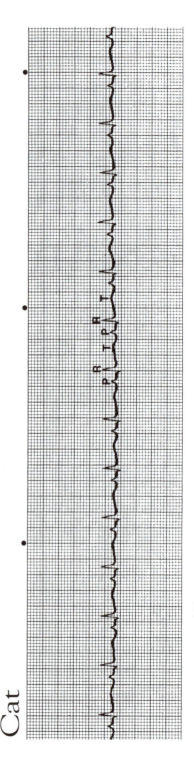

Cat

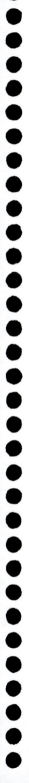

Normal Sinus Rhythm (NSR)

Sinus rhythm is the normal mechanism for initiating cardiac systole. The normal cardiac impulse originates in the sinoatrial node and spreads to the atria, the atrioventricular node, and the ventricles.

ECG Features

✓ The rhythm is regular at 70-160 bpm in dogs and 120-240 bpm in cats.

✓ There is less than 10% variation in the R-R intervals in dogs.

✓ In cats, the difference between the largest and the smallest R-R intervals is less than 0.10 sec.

➤ P waves are positive in lead II.

➤ P-QRS complexes are normal with a constant P-R interval.

✓ QRS complexes may be wide and bizarre if an intraventricular conduction defect is present.

Associated Conditions

✓ The sinus rhythm is the normal rhythm of the heart.

✓ Failure of the rhythm to meet any of the above criteria indicates the possible presence of some abnormality of impulse formation and/or impulse conduction, i.e. an *arrhythmia*.

Treatment

✓ No specific therapy is required.

Sinus Arrhythmia

Dog

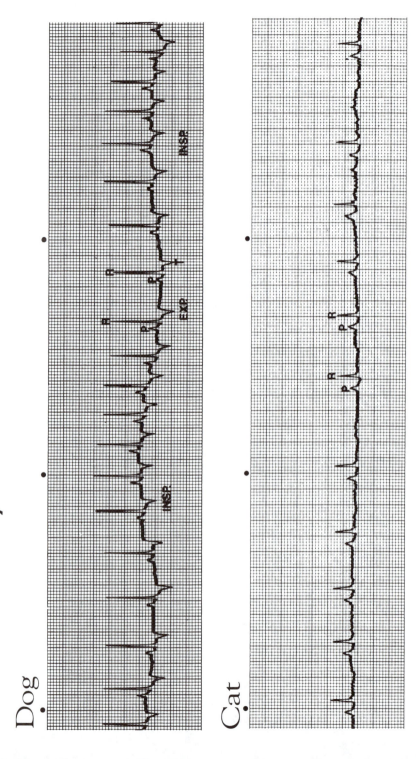

Cat

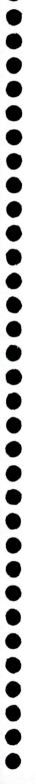

Sinus Arrhythmia (SA)

Sinus Arrhythmia (SA) is an irregular sinus rhythm originating in the sinoatrial node. It is represented by alternating periods of slower and more rapid heart rates usually related to respiration, the heart rate increasing with inspiration and decreasing with expiration. A nonrespiratory SA has no relationship to respiration.

ECG Features

❥ All criteria of normal sinus rhythm are met, except that the variation of R-R intervals is greater than 10%.

✓ The P wave, QRS complexes, and P-R intervals are normal.

✓ A wandering pacemaker (P waves varying in configuration), a variant of SA, is often present.

Associated Conditions

✓ Respiratory SA is a frequent normal finding in the dog.

✓ Respiratory SA is often seen in brachycephalic breeds or in chronic respiratory diseases, in which vagal tone is increased by upper airway obstruction.

✓ SA is accentuated by vagotonic procedures: carotid sinus and eyeball pressure and administration of digitalis.

✓ Atropine eliminates SA, indicating that its origin is vagal in nature.

Treatment

✓ No specific therapy is required.

Sinus Bradycardia

Dog

Cat

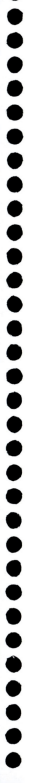

Sinus Bradycardia

is regular sinus rhythm, with a heart rate below normal discharge rates. Heart rates of 60-70 bpm may be normal for large breed dogs. In cats, it is often associated with a serious underlying disorder, which warrants attention and treatment.

ECG Features

◆ All criteria of normal sinus rhythm except that the heart rate is <70 bpm in dogs (<60 bpm in giant breeds) and <120 bpm in cats.

✓ The rhythm is regular, with a slight variation in R-R interval.

✓ P-R interval is constant.

Associated Conditions

✓ Physiologic: an increased vagal tone due to vomiting, intubation, elevated intracranial pressure; hypothermia, hypothyroidism, good conditioning, or respiratory disease.

✓ Pathologic: systemic disease with toxicity (e.g., renal failure), cardiac arrest. (Sinus bradycardia can be a warning of an impending cardiac arrest during surgery.)

✓ Drugs: phenothiazines, propranolol, digitalis, quinidine, morphine, and anesthetics, and calcium channel blockers.

✓ Central nervous system lesions.

✓ Hyperkalemia.

Treatment

✓ Treatment is rarely required.

✓ If clinical signs exist (weakness or collapse), atropine or glycopyrrolate should be administered IV followed by continuous IV infusion of isoproterenol or dobutamine if atropine is not helpful. Pro-Banthine may be used for long-term management. Theophylline or terbutaline may help to speed up heart rate.

✓ Right atrial pacing with a transvenous-pacing catheter is effective.

Sinus Tachycardia

Dog

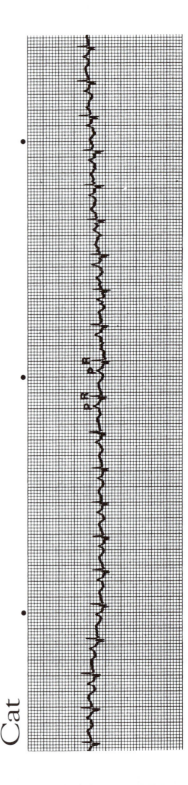

Cat

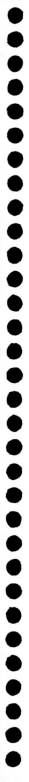

Sinus Tachycardia is regular sinus rhythm, with a heart rate above normal discharge rates.

Ocular pressure produces only a gradual transient slowing of the heart rate if any change at all.

ECG Features

◆ Acceleration of the sinoatrial node beyond its normal discharge rate, resulting in a heart rate >160 bpm in dogs (180 in toy breeds, 220 in puppies, and 140 in giant breeds) and >240 bpm in cats.

✓ The rhythm is regular, possibly with a slight variation in R-R interval.

✓ P-R interval is constant.

Associated Conditions

✓ Most common arrhythmia in dogs and cats.

✓ Physiologic: exercise, pain or restraint procedures (such as ECG recording).

✓ Pathologic: fever, hyperthyroidism, shock, anemia, infection, congestive heart failure, hypoxia.

✓ Drugs: atropine, epinephrine, vasodilators (hypotension).

✓ Hexachlorophene poisoning, electrical cord shock.

Treatment

✓ Treatment simply consists of identifying and controlling the causes. If the tachycardia is due to excitement, a tranquilizer will slow the heart rate; if it is due to congestive heart failure, digoxin for the underlying cardiac insufficiency is indicated.

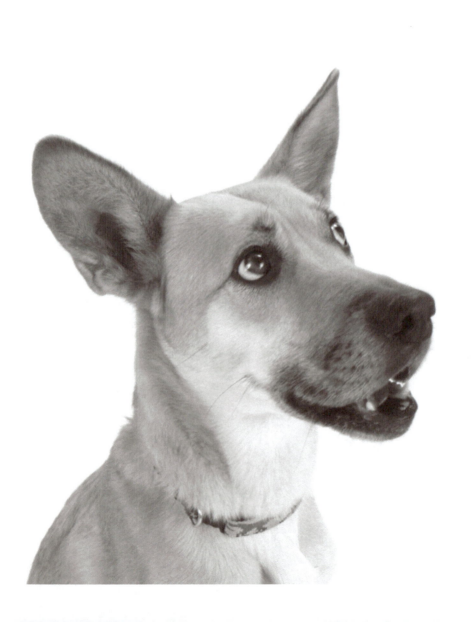

Section 2
Electro-cardiographic Examples

Disturbances of Supraventricular Impulse Formation

- ✓ Atrial Premature Complexes
- ✓ Atrial Tachycardia
- ✓ Atrial Fibrillation
- ✓ Atrioventricular Junctional Premature Complexes
- ✓ Atrioventricular Junctional Tachycardia

Atrial Premature Complexes

Dog

Cat

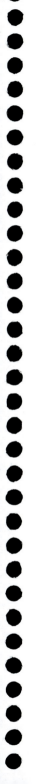

Atrial Premature Complexes (APCs)

are caused by supraventricular impulses originating from an ectopic atrial site (other than SA node). An increase in automaticity of atrial myocardial fibers or a single reentrant circuit are mechanisms for this arrhythmia.

ECG Features

❥ The heart rate is usually normal, and the rhythm is irregular due to the premature ectopic P wave that disrupts the normal P wave rhythm.

✓ In the P-QRS relationship the ectopic PR interval is usually as long as or longer than the sinus PR interval.

✓ The related QRS complex is usually of normal configuration (same as that of sinus complexes).

✓ The ectopic P wave has a different shape from that of the sinus P waves. It may be negative, positive biphasic, or superimposed on the previous T wave.

✓ A pause usually follows the APC. The ectopic atrial impulse discharges the sinus node and resets the cycle.

✱● APCs are easy to miss because they look just like normally conducted beats. Train your eye to look for P waves that unexpectedly touch the T wave of the previous beat. That, combined with the pause that follows the QRS-T, should help you catch them. APCs are the precursors to atrial tachycardia and atrial fibrillation, so it is important to identify them.

Associated Conditions

✓ Seen in dogs and cats, usually with atrial enlargement (e.g., mitral insufficiency, cardiomyopathy).

Treatment

Dogs–digoxin is often the treatment of choice. Treat any underlying congestive heart failure with appropriate dosage of diuretic and angiotensin converting enzyme inhibitor.

Cats–with hypertrophic cardiomyopathy use diltiazem or atenolol. Use digoxin for cats with dilated cardiomyopathy.

45

Atrial Tachycardia

Dog

Cat

Atrial Tachycardia

is a rapid regular rhythm originating from an atrial site other than the sinus node. Three or more APCs are considered to be atrial tachycardia. An abnormal automatic focus in the atrium is one cause. Another mechanism is reentry, a circuit between the atrium and AV junctional area, which allows the impulse to restimulate the atrium and pass to the ventricles.

ECG Features

✓ The heart rate is rapid (dogs, >160-180 bpm; cats, >240 bpm).

✓ Atrial tachycardia may be either intermittent (paroxysmal) or continuous.

✓ Configuration of the P waves is generally somewhat different than that of the sinus P waves. They may not be easy to see because of the fast ventricular rate or prolonged P-R interval.

✓ The QRS configuration is usually normal (same as the sinus complexes) or wide and bizarre because of bundle branch block or ventricular pre-excitation.

✓ The P-R interval is usually constant. At very high rates various degrees of AV block can occur.

Associated Conditions

✓ Commonly seen in dogs with severe heart disease and in cats with cardiomyopathy or hyperthyroidism.

✓ Associated with Wolff-Parkinson-White syndrome (congenital in cats and dogs).

✓ Same signalment as animals with APCs, those causing atrial enlargement being the most common.

Treatment

Dogs–Vagal maneuver (mild ocular or carotid sinus pressure) may effectively terminate reentrant atrial tachycardia. Intravenous esmolol, adenosine, verapamil, diltiazem, or digoxin may be administered slowly. Digoxin and diltiazem, or digoxin and propranolol or atenolol can be administered orally in combination. Quinidine gluconate has been used in isolated cases.

Cats–Diltiazem, atenolol, or digoxin.

Atrial Fibrillation
Dog

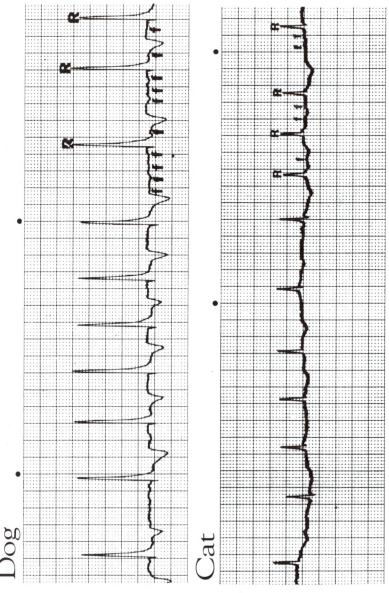

Cat

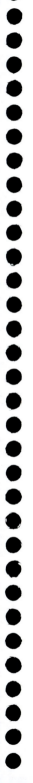

Atrial Fibrillation is caused by numerous disorganized atrial impulses frequently bombarding the AV node.

ECG Features

◆ Atrial fibrillation has a rapid and totally irregular atrial and ventricular rate. The ventricular rate is irregular because the atrioventricular junction allows only a limited number of fibrillatory waves to be conducted to the ventricles.

◆ Normal P waves are replaced by oscillations (f waves).

✓ The QRS configuration is normal (same as the sinus configuration) or wide and bizarre due to bundle branch block or ventricular pre-excitation.

✓ Normal QRS complexes often vary in amplitude.

Associated Conditions

✓ Commonly seen in dogs and cats with conditions associated with atrial enlargement, or dilated cardiomyopathy. Atrial fibrillation may occur in the absence of cardiac disease.

Treatment

Dogs–Treat the underlying congestive heart failure or other causes. To reduce the heart rate to less than 160 beats/min, digoxin is administered, followed by propranolol or diltiazem if additional slowing of the ventricular rate is necessary. Electrical cardioversion with precordial shock is indicated only when a rapid ventricular rate is unresponsive to drugs and when clinical signs exist.

Cats–with hypertrophic cardiomyopathy use diltiazem or atenolol. If the heart rate remains high add digoxin.

Atrioventricular (AV) Junctional Premature Complexes & Tachycardia

Dog

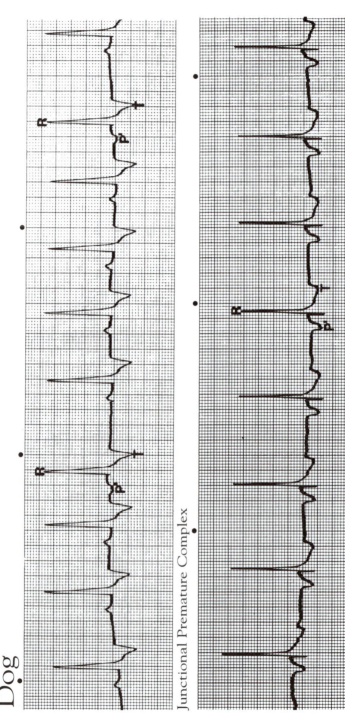

Junctional Premature Complex

Junctional Tachycardia

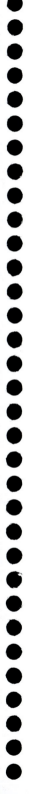

AV Junctional Premature Complexes—

are caused by the premature firing of an ectopic atrioventricular junctional focus. The impulse spreads backward (retrograde) to the atria, generating a negative P wave, as well as forward (anterograde) to the ventricles, generating a normal QRS complex. Because we cannot distinguish between a junctional focus and a low atrial ectopic focus, the term supraventricular is often preferred.

AV Junctional Tachycardia—

occurs when a junctional premature complex takes over as the primary pacemaker of the heart. The heart rate must be faster than the inherent canine atrioventricular junctional rate of 40-60 bpm. Sometimes termed supraventricular tachycardia.

ECG Features

Junctional Premature Complexes—

✓ Heart rate is usually normal, but the rhythm is irregular because of the premature P waves that disrupt normal P wave rhythm.

► P wave is almost always negative on lead II. P wave may precede, be superimposed on, or follow the QRS depending on the location of the ectopic focus.

✓ QRS complex is premature with a normal configuration (same as the sinus complexes) or wide and bizarre if bundle branch block, or ventricular pre-excitation is present.

✓ A noncompensatory pause is usually present.

*Junctional Tachycardia—*can be either paroxysmal (short bursts), or continuous. In the dog, the heart rate is over 60 bpm, with a regular rhythm. Complexes same as junctional premature complexes noted above.

Associated Conditions

✓ Digitalis toxicity.
✓ Same conditions that cause atrial premature contractions (APCs).

Treatment

✓ Treatment is the same as for APCs. If digitalis toxicity exists, discontinue the drug.

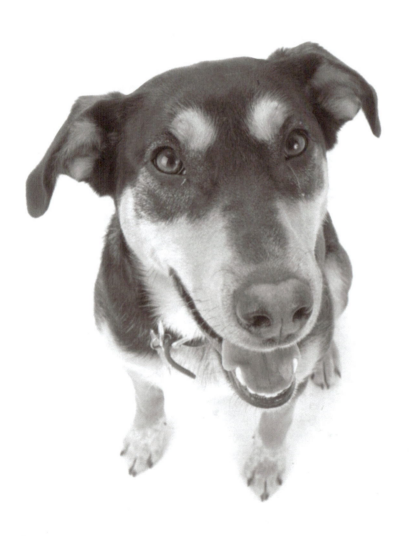

Section 2
Electro-
cardiographic
Examples

Disturbances of Ventricular Impulse Formation

- ✓ Ventricular Premature Complexes
- ✓ Ventricular Tachycardia
- ✓ Ventricular Asystole
- ✓ Ventricular Fibrillation

Ventricular Premature Complexes

Dog

Cat

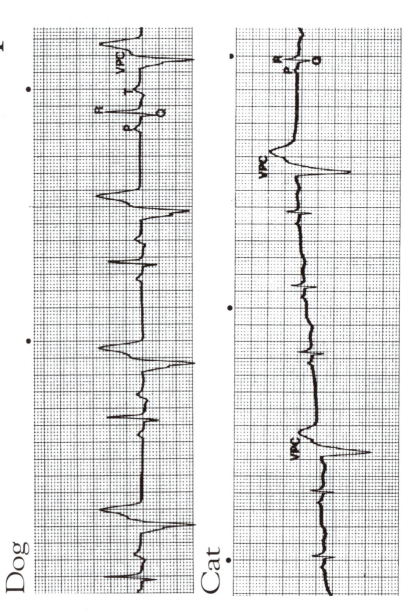

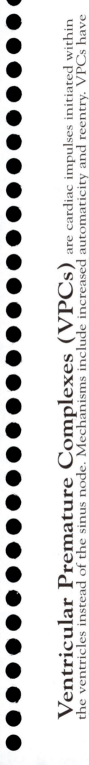

Ventricular Premature Complexes (VPCs) are cardiac impulses initiated within

the ventricles instead of the sinus node. Mechanisms include increased automaticity and reentry. VPCs have direct effects on the cardiovascular system with secondary effects on other systems because of poor perfusion. VPCs are associated with weakness, exercise intolerance, syncope, and sudden death.

ECG Features

❥ The QRS complexes are typically wide and bizarre.

❥ P waves are dissociated from the QRS complexes.

✓ A VPC is usually followed by a compensatory pause.

Associated Conditions

✓ Commonly seen in large breed dogs with cardiomyopathy, especially boxers and Doberman pinschers.

✓ Common in cats with cardiomyopathy; occasionally seen in cats with hyperthyroidism.

✓ Also seen with congenital defects (especially aortic stenosis), chronic valve disease, gastric torsion/volvulus, traumatic myocarditis (dogs), digitalis toxicity, cardiac neoplasia, and myocarditis.

Treatment

✓ Treatment of the asymptomatic patient is controversial. For the symptomatic patient restrict activity until the arrhythmia is controlled.

Dogs–procainamide, quinidine, tocainide, or mexiletine. Combine previous drugs with a beta-blocker if important arrhythmia persists. Consider sotalol or amiodarone as last resorts.

Cats–propranolol or atenolol are the preferred drugs.

Ventricular Tachycardia

Dog

Cat

Ventricular Tachycardia

is three or more VPCs in a row resulting from stimulation of an ectopic ventricular focus. Ventricular tachycardia may be intermittent (paroxysmal) or sustained. Potentially life threatening arrhythmia, usually signifying important myocardial disease or metabolic derangement. Direct effects are on the cardiovascular system, with secondary effects on other systems because of poor perfusion.

ECG Features

◆ The ventricular rate is >150 bpm with a regular rhythm. Ventricular Tachycardia between 60-100 bpm is termed idioventricular rhythm.

◆ QRS complexes are wide and bizarre. Ventricular fusion and capture complexes occur commonly with ventricular tachycardia.

◆ There is no relationship between the QRS complexes and the P waves. The P waves may precede, be hidden within, or follow the QRS complexes.

Associated Conditions

✓ Commonly seen in large-breed dogs with cardiomyopathy, especially boxers and Doberman pinschers.

✓ Uncommon in cats

✓ Other associated conditions are the same as those for VPCs.

Treatment

✓ Therapy should begin as soon as possible.

Dogs—lidocaine (IV boluses followed by infusion) is the treatment of choice. If lidocaine fails, administer IV procainamide to convert to sinus rhythm. When stable, start oral procainamide, quinidine, tocainide, or mexiletine. Combine previous drugs with a beta-blocker if arrhythmia persists. Treat underlying congestive heart failure with appropriate dosage of diuretic, angiotensin converting enzyme inhibitor, and vasodilator.

Cats—Propranolol or atenolol is preferred in cats. Use lidocaine cautiously and only for sustained ventricular tachycardia.

Ventricular Asystole

Dog

Cat

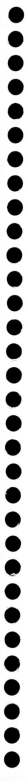

Ventricular Asystole

Ventricular Asystole indicates the absence of any pacemaker impulses. Subsequently, there is no depolarization or contraction of the ventricles. No pulse can be felt and cardiac output approaches zero, making this a life-threatening and generally terminal rhythm.

ECG Features

✓ P waves present if animal has complete atrioventricular block.

❥ No QRS complexes.

✓ Severe sinoatrial block or arrest.

Associated Conditions

✓ Any severe systemic illness (e.g., severe acidosis and hyperkalemia) or cardiac disease.

✓ Ventricular fibrillation and complete atrioventricular block.

✓ Electrical-mechanical dissociation represents a recorded ECG and no effective cardiac output.

Treatment

✓ Ventricular asystole is a rapid fatal rhythm requiring immediate, aggressive therapy.

✓ Institute CPR.

✓ Specific drugs of importance include epinephrine, atropine, and sodium bicarbonate.

✓ Treat any treatable problems such as hypothermia, hyperkalemia, and acid-base disorders.

✓ Artificial pacing with a transvenous pacemaker may be successful if myocardium is mechanically responsive.

✓ With electrical-mechanical dissociation, dopamine hydrochloride can be quite effective.

Ventricular Fibrillation

Dog

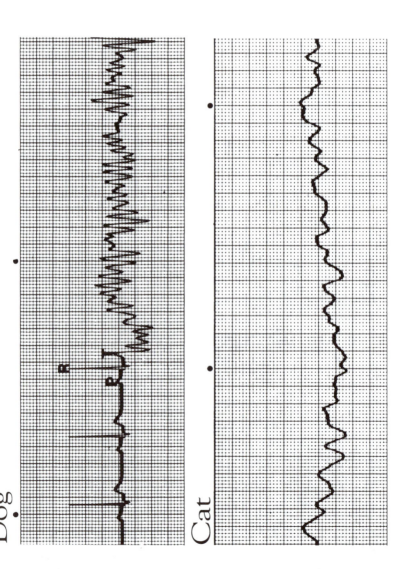

Cat

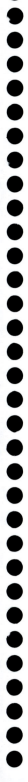

Ventricular Fibrillation occurs when the cells of the ventricular myocardium

depolarize in a chaotic and uncoordinated manner. No pulse can be felt and cardiac output approaches zero, making this a life-threatening and generally terminal rhythm.

ECG Features

❥ Rapid, chaotic, irregular rhythm with bizarre waves or oscillations.
❥ No QRS complexes or P waves.
✓ Oscillations may be large (coarse fibrillation) or small (fine fibrillation).

Associated Conditions

✓ History of severe systemic illness or cardiac disease in many animals or previous history of other cardiac arrhythmias.

✓ Shock, anoxia, trauma, myocardial infarction, electrolyte and acid-base imbalances, aortic stenosis, anesthetic reaction, digitalis toxicity, cardiac surgery, electrical shock, myocarditis, hypothermia, or autonomic effects.

Treatment

✓ Ventricular fibrillation is a rapid fatal rhythm requiring immediate, aggressive therapy. Patient will probably die without electrical cardioversion.

✓ Epinephrine may change fine fibrillation to coarse fibrillation and increase the chances of electrical cardioversion.

✓ Once converted, administer lidocaine to lower the risk of refibrillation or ventricular tachycardia.

✓ If no access to a defibrillator, attempt conversion with potassium and acetylcholine, and/or administer a precordial thump. Rarely successful, but you have nothing to lose.

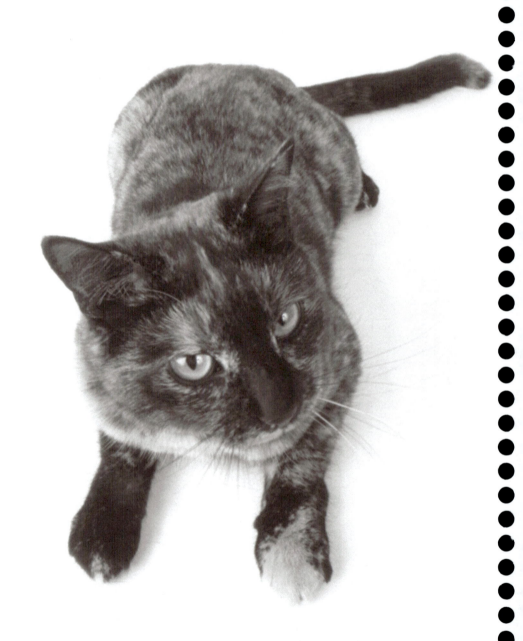

Section 2
Electro-cardiographic Examples

Disturbances of Impulse Conduction

- ✓ Sinus Arrest or Block
- ✓ Sick Sinus Syndrome
- ✓ Atrial Standstill
- ✓ Ventricular Pre-Excitation
- ✓ First-Degree Atrioventricular Block
- ✓ Second-Degree Atrioventricular Block
- ✓ Third-Degree Atrioventricular Block
- ✓ Left Bundle Branch Block
- ✓ Right Bundle Branch Block

Sinus Arrest or Block

Dog

Cat

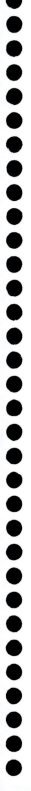

Sinus Arrest or Block

Sinus Arrest—normal sinus rhythm interrupted by an occasional, prolonged failure of the sinoatrial node to initiate an impulse. Sinus Block—conduction disturbance in which normal sinus rhythm is interrupted by an occasional, prolonged failure of the impulse generated by the sinoatrial node to reach the atria. With prolonged pauses, periods of low cardiac output may occur.

ECG Features

✓ The heart rate varies and is often correlated with bradycardia.

✓ Rhythm is regularly irregular or irregular with pauses.

✓ Normal P wave for each QRS complex.

❥ Pauses–two times the normal R-R interval.

Associated Conditions

✓ Normal incidental finding in brachycephalic breeds of dog.

❥ Seen in dog breeds predisposed to sick sinus syndrome.

✓ Seen in purebred pugs with hereditary stenosis of the bundle of His.

✓ Reported in dalmation coach hounds that are born deaf.

✓ Uncommon in cats.

✓ Vagal stimulation, coughing, pharyngeal irritation, carotid sinus massage, degenerative heart disease, irritation of vagus nerve secondary to thoracic or cervical neoplasia, neoplastic heart disease, electrolyte imbalance, and drug toxicity (e.g. digitalis, quinidine, and propranolol) are other causative factors for sinus block.

Treatment

✓ None if animal is asymptomatic.

❥ Treat underlying cause. An artificial pacemaker can be considered in animals unresponsive to treatment.

65

Sick Sinus Syndrome
Dog

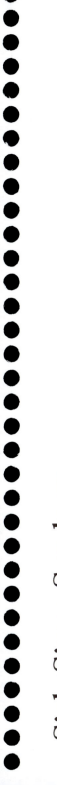

Sick Sinus Syndrome

Sick Sinus Syndrome is a term given to a number of ECG abnormalities of the sinoatrial (SA) node including severe sinus bradycardia and severe sinus block. Many cases with these ECG changes have recurrent episodes of supraventricular tachycardia in addition to the underlying slow sinus rhythm (bradycardia-tachycardia syndrome). The majority of sick sinus syndrome cases also have coexisting abnormalities of the atrioventricular (AV) junction and/or bundle branches. During the long periods of sinus block, the latent AV junctional pacemaker fails to pace the heart; the result is cardiac standstill.

ECG Features

✓ Severe and persisting sinus bradycardia not induced by drugs.

▶ Sinus block occurs with or without escape rhythms.

✓ In the bradycardia-tachycardia syndrome, there are periods of severe sinus bradycardia alternating with ectopic supraventricular tachycardias (atrial tachycardia, atrial fibrillation, or atrial flutter).

✓ Long pause following an atrial premature complex.

✓ AV junctional escape rhythm (with or without slow and unstable sinus activity).

✓ Atrial fibrillation with a slow ventricular rate in the absence of drugs is usually due to disease of the AV junction.

Associated Conditions

✓ Not identified in cats.

✓ Female miniature schnauzers of at least 6 years of age with a history of syncope and weakness.

✓ Disease affecting SA node artery or replacement of the SA node with fibrous tissue.

Treatment

▶ The treatment of choice is a permanent artificial pacemaker.

✓ If symptomatic, drug therapy (e.g., atropine, isoproterenol and digitalis) is usually not successful because the drug for treating the tachyarrhythmia aggravates the bradyarrhythmia and vice versa. Theophylline (long acting) can be useful to reduce the length of pauses (sinus block).

Atrial Standstill

Dog

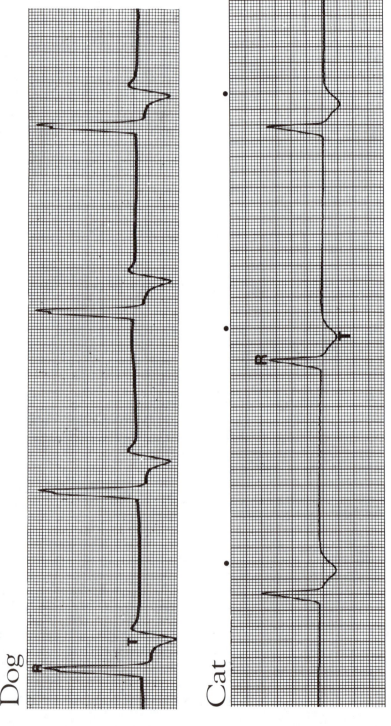

Cat

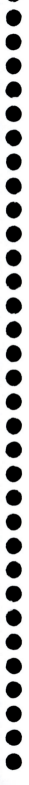

Atrial Standstill

Atrial Standstill is characterized by an absence of P waves and by a regular escape rhythm with a supraventricular-type QRS. Condition can be temporary (i.e., associated with hyperkalemia or drug induced), terminal (i.e., associated with severe hyperkalemia or dying heart), or persistent. Hyperkalemic patients with atrial standstill have sinus node function, but impulses do not cause atrial myocyte activation. Persistent atrial standstill is caused by inherited atrial myopathy.

ECG Features

✓ The heart rate is slow, <60 bpm and the rhythm is regular.

🖤 No P waves are observed in any lead.

✓ QRS complexes are usually normal if the animal has persistent atrial standstill or hyperkalemia and may be wide if the animal has severe hyperkalemia or bundle branch block.

Associated Conditions

✓ Hyperkalemia.

✓ Persistent atrial standstill—atrial myopathy is most common in English springer spaniels. Most affected animals are young. Skeletal muscle involvement is common.

✓ Atrial disease, often associated with atrial distention (cats with cardiomyopathy).

Treatment

🖤 Persistent atrial standstill—a permanent ventricular pacemaker should be implanted if the patient is symptomatic. Treat with diuretics, digoxin (after pacemaker implant), and ACE inhibitor if CHF develops.

✓ Temporary atrial standstill—Calcium gluconate counters the effects of hyperkalemia and can be used in life-threatening situations to reestablish a sinus rhythm while instituting treatment to lower potassium concentration (e.g., 0.9% saline, sodium bicarbonate, dextrose and/or regular insulin).

✓ Heart rate does not increase with atropine administration.

Ventricular Pre-excitation and Wolff-Parkinson-White Syndrome

Dog

Cat

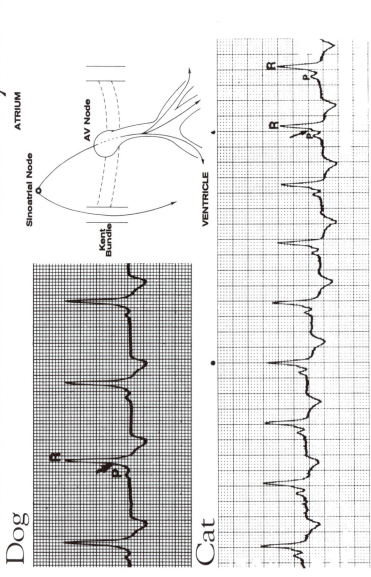

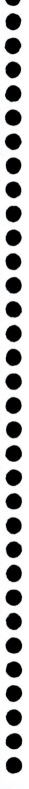

Ventricular Pre-excitation

Ventricular Pre-excitation occurs when impulses originating in the sinoatrial node or atrium activate a portion of the ventricles prematurely through the atrioventricular node. The remainder of the ventricles are activated normally through the usual conduction system. Wolff-Parkinson-White (WPW) syndrome consists of ventricular pre-excitation with episodes of paroxysmal supraventricular tachycardia.

ECG Features

✓ Normal heart rate and rhythm.

✓ Normal P waves.

✦ Short P-R interval (dogs, <0.06 sec; cats, <0.05 sec).

✦ Widened QRS (small dogs, >0.05 sec; large dogs, >0.06 sec; cats, >0.04 sec), often with a delta wave (slurring or notching of the upstroke of the R wave).

✓ Ventricular pre-excitation with WPW also has an extremely rapid heart rate (dogs >300 bpm, cats 400-500 bpm). Additionally, the QRS complexes may be normal, wide with delta wave, or very wide and bizarre depending on the circuit.

Associated Conditions

✓ Congenital defect limited to the conduction system.

✓ Atrial septal defect in dogs or cats.

✓ Tricuspid valvular dysplasia in dogs.

✓ Hypertrophic cardiomyopathy in cats.

Treatment

✓ Ventricular pre-excitation without tachycardia does not require treatment.

✓ WPW syndrome requires conversion by ocular or carotid sinus pressure, direct current shock (the most effective treatment), or drugs (dogs only—lidocaine bolus followed by IV drip or oral procainamide; cats or dogs—propranolol, atenolol, or diltiazem).

71

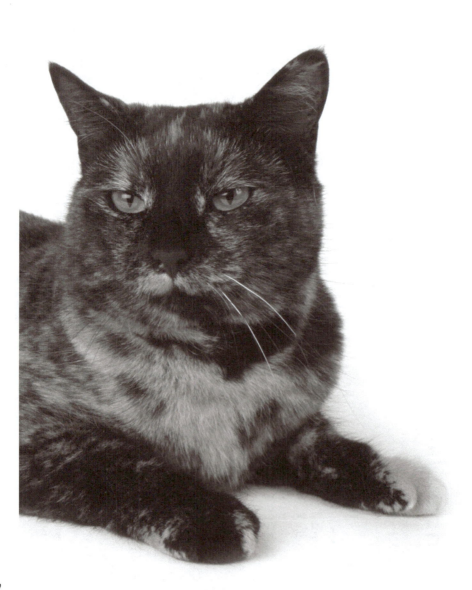

The Secret to Atrioventricular Blocks

First-Degree AV Block—
"All" of the beats go through the AV node
(but with delayed conduction)

Second-Degree AV Block—
"Some" of the beats go through

Third-Degree AV Block—
"None" of the beats go through

First-Degree Atrioventricular Block

Dog

Cat

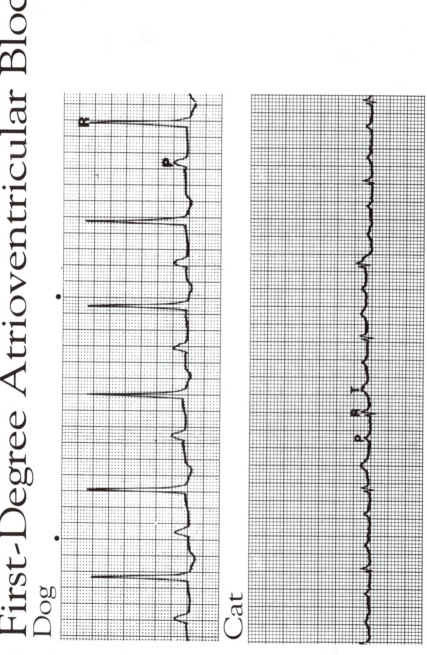

First-Degree Atrioventricular Block is a delay in conduction of a

supraventricular impulse through the atrioventricular junction and bundle of His.

ECG Features

✓ The rate and rhythm is usually normal.

✓ The P wave is normal.

✓ The QRS is usually normal.

➤ Prolongation of the P-R interval >.13 sec in dogs, >.09 sec in cats, in the presence of normal sinus rhythm.

Associated Conditions

✓ Generally seen in older patients secondary to degenerative changes in the conduction system.

✓ Common as an aging change in cocker spaniels and dachshunds.

✓ Patients are usually asymptomatic.

✓ Reflex vagal stimulation (generally results in cyclic increase in P-R interval).

✓ Drug therapy (e.g. digoxin, propranolol, quinidine, and procainamide). Low dosages of atropine initially prolong the P-R interval. If secondary to digoxin toxicity, may see signs of lethargy, anorexia, vomiting and diarrhea. Lengthening of the P-R interval should not be used as an indicator of digoxin serum concentration; 50% of digitalized dogs have a prolonged P-R interval.

✓ First-degree atrioventricular block may also be seen with potassium imbalance, hypothyroidism or protozoal myocarditis.

Treatment

✓ Treat any underlying cause.

✓ Recognize association with certain antiarrhythmic drugs.

Second-Degree Atrioventricular Block

Second-Degree Atrioventricular Block is characterized by an intermittent failure or disturbance of atrioventricular (AV) conduction. One or more P waves are not followed by QRS-T complexes. Second-degree atrioventricular block can be classified into two types: Mobitz type I (Wenkebach) and Mobitz type II. The classification can further be defined by QRS duration; and type B (lesion below the His bundle), with a wide QRS complex.

Dog

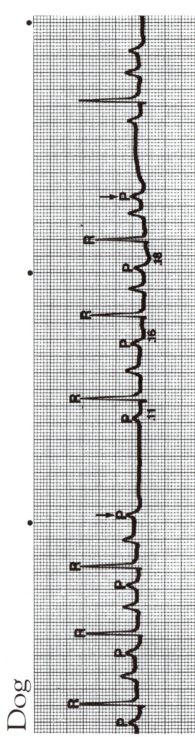

Mobitz I Type A

ECG Features of Second Degree AV Block–Mobitz Type I

❤ P waves can be seen that do not conduct QRS complexes.

✓ The P waves are normal and consistent appearing.

❤ The P-R interval is often variable. There may be progressive prolongation of the P-R interval with successive beats until a P wave is blocked.

✓ The QRS duration is normal. Mobitz type I is usually type A (block involves conduction failure above the bifurcation of the His bundle producing a normal duration QRS complex)

✓ The ventricular rate is slower than the atrial rate because of blocked P waves.

Second-Degree Atrioventricular Block (continued)

Dog

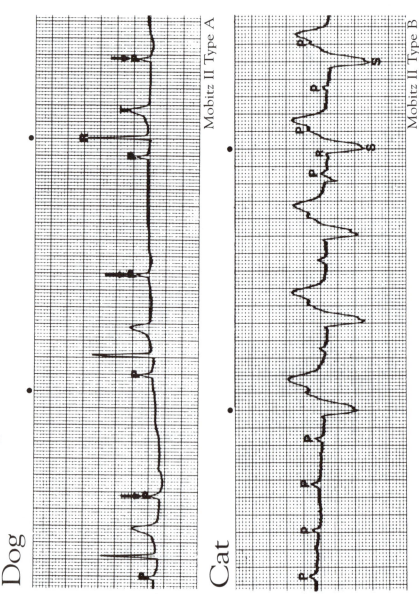

Mobitz II Type A

Cat

Mobitz II Type B

ECG Features of Second-Degree AV Block, Mobitz type II

✓ Mobitz type II is more serious than Mobitz type I because frequency and severity of the block is unpredictable.

➤ P waves can be seen that do not conduct QRS complexes. The P waves are normal and consistent appearing.

➤ The P-R intervals are constant (i.e., do not vary preceding a blocked beat).

✓ The QRS complexes are often of abnormal configuration. Mobitz type II is usually type B (block occurs below the bifurcation of the His bundle producing a wide QRS complex).

✓ Advanced second-degree AV block, Mobitz type II occurs when two or more consecutive P waves are blocked.

✓ A fixed relationship between the atria and ventricles may occur (i.e., 2:1, 3:1, and 4:1 AV block).

✓ The ventricular rate is slower than the atrial rate because of the blocked P waves.

Associated Conditions of Second-Degree AV Block

✓ May be a normal finding, especially in young dogs. Sinus arrhythmia and other causes of increased vagal tone.

✓ Supraventricular tachycardia.

✓ Microscopic idiopathic fibrosis in older dogs.

✓ Hereditary stenosis of the His bundle in Pugs.

✓ Hypertrophic cardiomyopathy or hyperthyroidism in cats.

✓ Myocarditis, including Lyme disease.

✓ Drug administration (e.g., digoxin, propranolol, diltiazem, and lidocaine). Electrolyte imbalances. Low doses of IV atropine. Xylazine as an anesthetic.

✓ Cardiac neoplasia.

Treatment

✓ For Mobitz type I (type A) treatment is usually not necessary.

✓ If wide QRS complexes occur with type B, treatment may be necessary. These cases have the tendency to develop third-degree atrioventricular block. Treatment may include atropine, glycopyrrolate, isoproterenol or artificial pacing. Correct any electrolyte abnormalities. Discontinue drugs that suppress AV conduction.

Third-Degree Atrioventricular Block
(Complete Block)

Dog

Cat

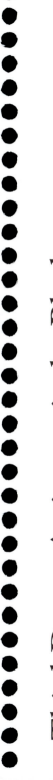

Third-Degree Atrioventricular Block

The cardiac impulse is completely blocked in the region of the atrioventricular (AV) junction and/or all bundle branches. The atrial rate (P-P interval) is normal. The idioventricular escape rhythm is slow.

ECG Features

◆ The ventricular rate is slower than the atrial rate (more P waves than QRS complexes). A ventricular escape rhythm usually has a rate of 40-60 in dogs and 60-100 in cats.

✓ The P wave is normal.

✓✓ The QRS is wide and bizarre when the pacemaker is located in the ventricle, or in the lower AV junction (above the bifurcation of the bundle of His) in a patient with bundle branch block.

✓ The QRS complex is normal when the escape pacemaker is located in the lower AV junction in a patient without bundle branch block.

◆ There is no conduction between the atria and ventricles. The P waves have no constant relationship with the QRS complexes. The P-P and R-R intervals are relatively constant (except for sinus arrhythmia).

Associated Conditions

✓ Isolated congenital defect or other congenital defects (aortic stenosis, ventricular septal defect).

✓ Severe digitalis toxicity (usually underlying cardiac pathology).

✓ Infiltrative cardiomyopathy: amyloidosis, neoplasia

✓ Idiopathic fibrosis, in older dogs, especially Cocker spaniels.

✓ Additional causes are hypertrophic cardiomyopathy, endocarditis, myocarditis, myocardial infarction, hyperkalemia, and Lyme disease.

Treatment

◆ A temporary or permanent cardiac pacemaker is usually the only effective treatment in symptomatic patients.

81

Left Bundle Branch Block

Dog

I | II | III | aVR | aVL | aVF

Cat

I | II | III | aVR | aVL | aVF

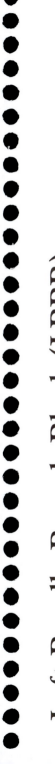

Left Bundle Branch Block (LBBB)

Conduction delay or block in both the left posterior and left anterior fascicles of the left bundle. A supraventricular impulse activates the right ventricle first through the right bundle branch. The left ventricle is then activated late, causing the QRS to become wide and bizarre.

ECG Features

❥ The QRS is prolonged (>0.08 sec in dogs; >0.06 in cats).

❥ The QRS is positive in leads I, II, III, and AVF.

✓ The block can be intermittent or constant.

Associated Conditions

✓ Uncommon in cats and dogs. Usually an incidental ECG finding.

✓ Severe underlying bundle branch disease (because the left bundle branch is thick and extensive, the lesion is required to be large). The lesion causing the block could progress, leading to more serious arrhythmias or complete heart block.

✓ Direct or indirect cardiac trauma (e.g. hit by car and cardiac needle puncture).

✓ Neoplasia.

✓ Congenital defect (subvalvular aortic stenosis).

✓ Fibrosis.

✓ Cardiomyopathy.

✓ Ischemic cardiomyopathy (e.g. arteriosclerosis of the coronary arteries, myocardial infarction, and myocardial hypertrophy which obstructs coronary arteries).

Treatment

✓ Treatment should be directed toward the underlying cause. LBBB does not cause hemodynamic abnormalities.

83

Right Bundle Branch Block

Dog

I	II	III	aVR	aVL	aVF

Cat

I	II	III	aVR	aVL	aVF

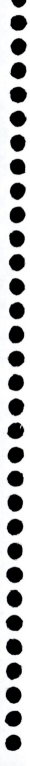

Right Bundle Branch Block (RBBB)

Conduction delay or block in the right bundle branch resulting in late activation of the right ventricle. The block can be complete or incomplete.

ECG Features

✓ A right axis deviation and wide QRS (>0.08 sec in dogs; >0.06 in cats) in most animals.
❧ Large, wide S-waves in leads I, II, III, and AVF.

Associated Conditions

❧ Occasionally seen in normal and healthy dogs and cats. Usually an incidental ECG finding.
✓ In beagles, incomplete RBBB can be a genetically determined localized variation in right ventricular wall thickness.
✓ Congenital heart disease.
✓ Chronic valvular fibrosis.
✓ After surgical correction of a cardiac defect.
✓ Trauma caused by cardiac needle puncture to obtain blood sample or trauma from other causes.
✓ Chronic infection with Chagas' disease.
✓ Cardiac neoplasia.
✓ Heartworm disease.
✓ Acute thromboembolism.
✓ Cardiomyopathy.
✓ Hyperkalemia (most commonly in cats with urethral obstruction).

Treatment

✓ Treatment should be directed toward the underlying cause.

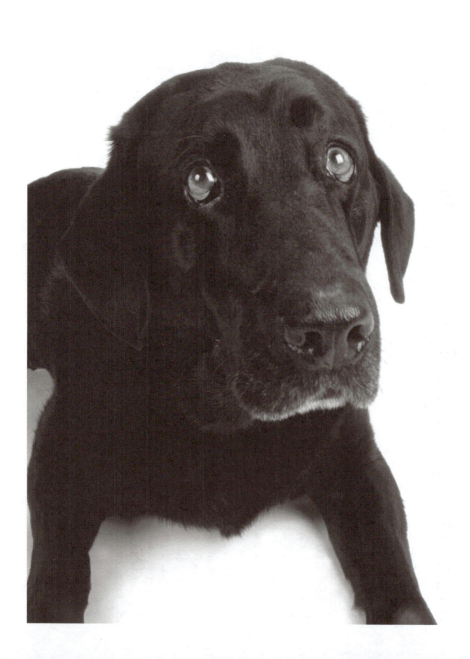

Section 2
Electro-cardiographic Examples

Escape Rhythms

✓ Junctional Escape Rhythms
✓ Ventricular Escape Rhythms

Escape Rhythms
Dog

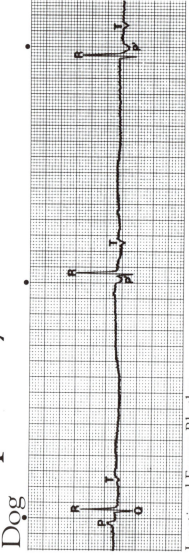

Junctional Escape Rhythm

Cat

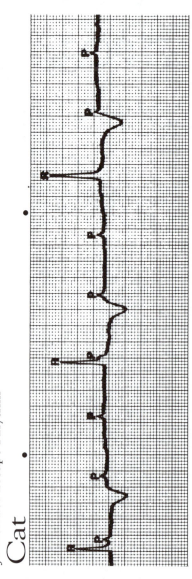

Ventricular Escape Rhythm with Complete AV Block

Escape Rhythms

occur when the pacemaker with the highest automaticity (usually the sinoatrial node) either slows down or stops. The intrinsic pacemaker activity of the lower regions of the heart, the atrioventricular (AV) junction or the ventricles, rescues the heart rhythm after a pause in the dominant rhythm. If the subsidiary pacemaker temporarily takes over the role of the cardiac pacemaker, the rhythm is known as an escape rhythm.

ECG Features of Junctional & Ventricular (Idioventricular) Escape Rhythms

The heart rate is slow. Escape complexes follow a pause longer than the normal sinus cycle length (R-R interval). Rhythm is regular when the escape rhythm is dominant.

Junctional Escape Rhythm—

✓ The P wave is usually negative and may precede, be superimposed on, or follow the QRS complex; and the QRS configuration is usually normal.

Ventricular Escape Rhythm—

✓ The P waves are not present, unless complete AV block or high-grade second-degree AV block exists (P waves will then be unrelated to, precede, be hidden within, or follow the ectopic QRS complexes).

✓ The QRS configuration is wide and bizarre, similar to that of premature ventricular contractions. No relationship exists between the P waves and QRS complexes.

Associated Conditions

✓ All the causes of sinus bradycardia and AV block.

Treatment

● Treat the underlying cause of the arrhythmia because the escape rhythm is a secondary phenomenon. The actual escape rhythm should not be treated, as it is a safety mechanism for maintaining cardiac output.

✓ Atropine or glycopyrrolate. Artificial pacing if the arrhythmia is resistant to drug treatment. Causative drugs, such as, digoxin, propranolol, or anesthetics, should be discontinued.

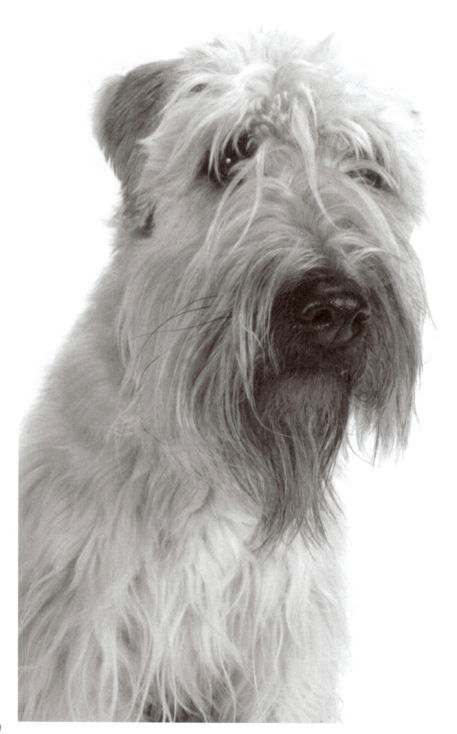

Section 2
Electro-cardiographic Examples

Miscellaneous Disturbances

- ✓ Pericardial Effusion (low voltage QRS complexes and electrical alternans)
- ✓ ST Segment and T Wave Changes
- ✓ Artifacts

Pericardial Effusion (Low Voltage QRS Complexes & Electrical Alternans)

Dog

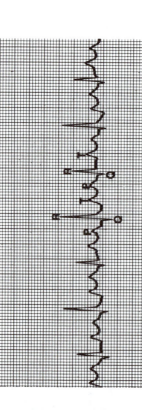

Electrical alternans and low amplitudes in a dog with pericardial effusion.

Cat

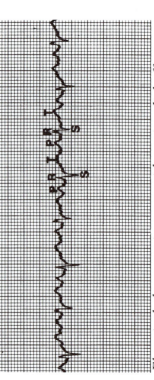

Electrical alternans in a cat with pericardial effusion.

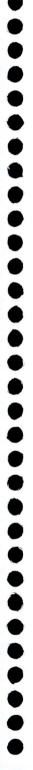

Low Voltage QRS Complexes & Electrical Alternans

Pericardial effusion is a common cause of low-amplitude complexes and electrical alternans (complexes that are regular but alternate in height or direction).

ECG Features

Low voltage QRS complexes—low amplitude complexes in all leads (<0.5 mV on lead II in the dog).
Electrical alternans—QRS complexes alternate in height or direction.

Associated Conditions

Low voltage QRS complexes—

➤ Normal variation, obesity, or incorrect standardization.

➤ Pericardial or pleural effusion.

➤ Hypothyroidism.

➤ Pulmonary edema, emphysema, or pneumonia.

➤ Myocardial damage, e.g., myocardial infarction, cardiomyopathy (infiltrative neoplasm, myocardial fibrosis).

➤ Cardiomyopathy after adriamycin chemotherapy.

➤ Pneumothorax.

Electrical alternans—

➤ Pericardial effusion: heart base tumors or metastatic carcinoma, right-sided heart failure, benign idiopathic pericardial effusion.

➤ Bundle branch block or supraventricular tachycardia.

Treatment

➤ Electrical alternans in pericardial effusion usually indicates a large effusion with possible cardiac tamponade. Pericardiocentesis is often indicated. Treatment should be directed at the underlying disorder, if one is present.

ST Segment & T Wave Changes

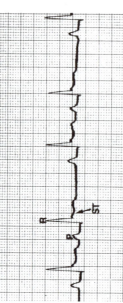

ST segment depression in a cat with hypertrophic cardiomyopathy.

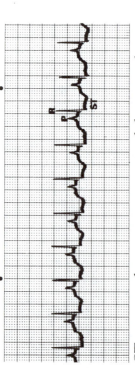

ST segment coving (arrow) in a dog with left bundle branch block.

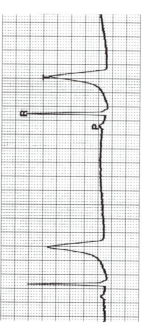

ST segment elevation (arrow) from myocardial hypoxia in a dog during surgery.

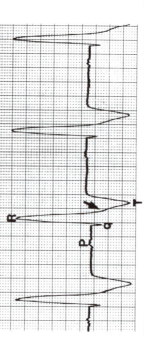

Tall, narrow, and pointed T waves of hyperkalemia (K+, 6.2 mEq/L) in a dog.

A word of advice: Don't get too hung up on S-T segment and T wave abnormalities. They can be helpful additional information but specific diagnoses cannot always be linked to them.

ST Segment

—represents the time from the end of the QRS complex to the onset of the T wave, (i.e., the early phase of ventricular repolarization). It may be elevated, at, or depressed from the level of the baseline. The baseline (isoelectric line) is the segment just prior to the P wave.

T Wave

—is the first major deflection following the QRS complex. It represents the recovery period of the ventricles and may be positive, notched, negative, or diphasic. It may be of abnormal amplitude, shape or direction.

ECG Features

S-T segment—marked and consistent elevation or depression of the S-T segment compared to baseline.
T wave—should not be greater than 25% of the R wave amplitude. The T wave should remain a constant shape on a given lead for the animal's lifetime. Therefore, a marked change in shape or polarity in the T wave on serial ECGs is usually abnormal.

Associated Conditions

S-T segment—
✓ Normal variation.
✓ S-T segment depression (myocardial ischemia, myocardial infarction, hyperkalemia, hypokalemia, digitalis toxicity, trauma to the heart).
✓ S-T segment elevation (myocardial infarction, pericarditis, myocardial hypoxia).
✓ Secondary S-T segment changes following abnormalities of the QRS complex (hypertrophy, bundle branch block, and ventricular premature complexes).
T wave—myocardial hypoxia, bundle branch blocks or ventricular enlargement, electrolyte imbalances, metabolic diseases, drug toxicity, and respiratory abnormalities.

Treatment

—should be directed to the underlying disorder, if one is present.

95

Artifacts

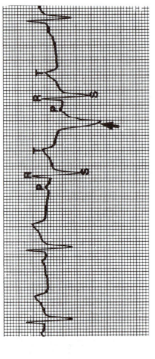

Movement artifact (arrow) from dog jerking its leg.

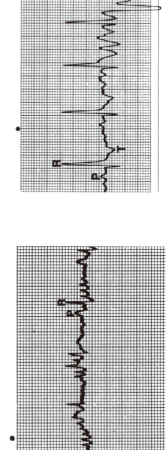

Trembling artifact simulating atrial and/or ventricular arrhythmias.

Electrical interference (60-cycle).

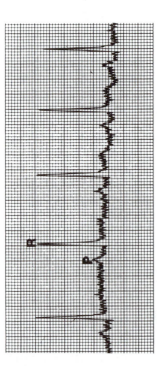

Purring artifact (arrow) from a cat.

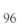

Technical Recording Problems

✓ Lead reversal, incorrect electrode placement, is a common error that can simulate right-sided enlargement.

✓ If standardization is improperly labeled, voltages may appear abnormally low or high.

✓ For measurement purposes standard paper speed is 50 mm/sec. If the tracing is run at 25 mm/sec and you think it is at 50 mm/sec, false measurements will result.

✓ Electrical interference, 60-cycle artifact, is due to improper grounding.

✓ A poorly defined baseline indicates a dirty stylus or low stylus heat.

✓ Common problems with electrodes and cables include: broken cable, loose connection of the alligator clip to the cable tip, dirty cable tips, cable wires pulling on the electrodes, or a swinging cable over the table edge.

Animal-Related Factors

✓ Artifacts can result from muscle tremor or from unexpected animal body movements.

✓ A wandering baseline, often from respiratory movements, coughing, or voluntary motion by the animal or handler, can simulate atrial and ventricular arrhythmias.

So how do we tell artifact from arrhythmias?

✓ The most important realization is that artifacts do not interrupt atrial or ventricular rhythm.

✓ The rhythm of artifacts is usually irregular and the rate of artifacts is usually variable.

97

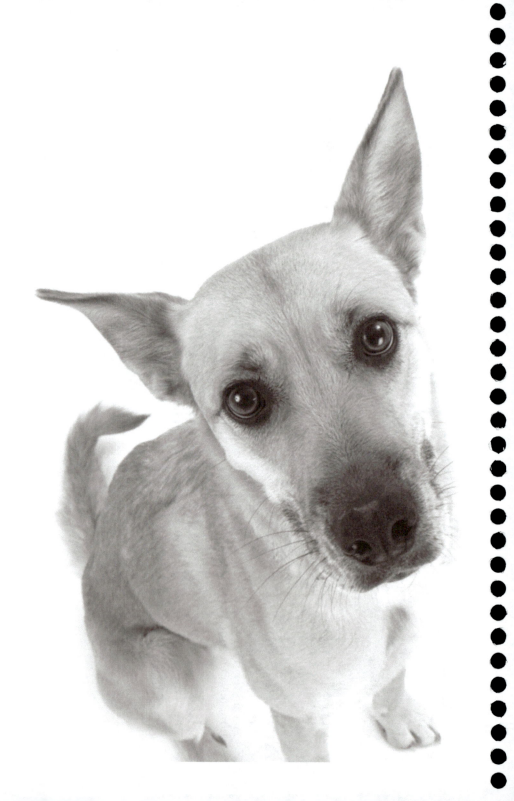

Appendix

Anti-Arrhythmic Drugs

Recommended
Textbook Readings

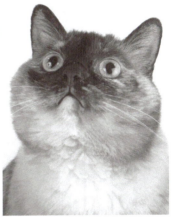

Anti-Arrhythmic Drugs

Drug	Formulation	Indications	Dog Dose (D) / Cat Dose (C)	Comments
Atenolol (Tenormin)	Tab: 25, 50, 100 mg Inj: 0.5 mg/ml in 10 ml ampules	Atrial and ventricular arrhythmias, hypertrophic cardiomyopathy, hypertension	D: 0.25-1.0 mg/kg PO q 12-24 h C: 6.25-12.5 mg/cat PO q 24 h	Less bronchoconstriction, vaso-constriction, and interference with insulin therapy than with nonselective agents Taper dose when discontinuing therapy Decrease dose with renal disease
Atropine sulfate	Inj: 0.05, 0.1, 0.3, 0.4, 0.5, 0.8, 1.0 mg/ml	Sinus bradycardia, AV block, sick sinus syndrome, cardiac arrest	D: 0.01-0.04 mg/kg IV, IM, IO 0.02-0.04 mg/kg, q 6-8 h SC (IT: double dose) C: Same	May transiently worsen bradyarrhythmia More potent chronotropic effects than glycopyrrolate
Digoxin (Cardoxin, Lanoxin)	Tab: 0.125, 0.25, 0.5 mg Inj: 0.25 mg/ml Elixir: 0.05 mg/ml, 0.15 mg/ml Cap: 0.05, 0.1, 0.2 mg	Supraventricular arrhythmias, myocardial failure	D: *Maintenance dose:* 0.22 mg/M^2 q 12 h PO 0.0055-0.01 mg/kg q 12 h PO *IV loading dose:* 0.02 mg/kg IV, 1/4 q 1 hr to effect Begin oral therapy 12 hours later *Oral loading dose:* Twice the maintenance dose for the first 24-48 hours C: 2-4 kg: 1/4 of 0.125 mg tab q 48 h 4-6 kg: 1/4 of 0.125 mg tab q 24-48 h >6 kg: 1/4 of 0.125 mg tab q 12 h	Toxicity potentiated by hypokalemia, hypomagnesemia, hyponatremia, hypercalcemia, thyroid disorders, hypoxia Dose on lean body weight, reduce dose 10-15% with elixirs Therapeutic range 1-2 ng/ml; 8-10 hours after a dose Rapid digitalization not recommended except in emergency Reduce dose 50% with quinidine
Diltiazem (Cardizem, Dilacor)	Tab: 30, 60, 90, 120 mg Capsules (Cardizem CD): 120, 180, 240, 300 mg Capsules (Dilacor): 180, 240 mg Inj: 5 mg/ml in 25 and 50 mg vials	Supraventricular arrhythmias, hypertrophic cardiomyopathy, hypertension	D: 0.5-1.5 mg/kg q 8 h PO (titrate to effect) 0.25 mg/kg slowly IV C: 1.5-2.5 mg/kg q 8 h PO Cardizem CD: 10 mg/kg q 24 h PO Dilacor: 5-10 mg/kg q 24 h PO 0.25 mg/kg slowly IV	Less myocardial depression than verapamil Cardizem CD capsules need to be compounded for use in cats

Drug	Formulations	Indications	Dosage	Comments
Epinephrine (Adrenalin)	Inj: 1:1000 conc (1 mg/ml) 1:10,000 conc (0.1 mg/ml)	Cardiac arrest	D: 0.2 mg/kg IV, IO q 3-5 min Double doses for IT administration C: Same	Monitor with ECG Previously recommended dose of 0.02 mg/kg may be a safer starting dose if a defibrillator is not available
Isoproterenol (Isuprel)	Inj: 1:5000 (0.2 mg/ml)	Short-term management of sinus bradycardia, AV block, sick sinus syndrome	D: 0.04-0.09 μg/kg/min IV (titrate to effect) 0.1-0.2 mg q 4-6 h IM, SC C: Same	
Lidocaine (Xylocaine)	Inj: 5, 10, 15, 20 mg/ml (without epinephrine)	Ventricular arrhythmias	D: 2-8 mg/kg slowly IV or IO (double the dose IT) in 2 mg/kg boluses followed by IV drip at 25-75 (occasionally up to 100) μg/kg/min CRI C: 0.25-0.75 mg/kg IV over 5 min	Use with caution in cats Drug of choice for initial control of ventricular tachycardia Effects increased by high potassium and decreased by low potassium Seizures controlled with diazepam Do not use formulations with epinephrine for arrhythmia control
Mexiletine (Mexitil)	Cap: 150, 200, 250 mg	Ventricular arrhythmias	D: 5-8 mg/kg q 8 h PO C: none	Reduce dose with liver disease Take with food to reduce GI side effects
Procainamide (Procan SR, Pronestyl)	Cap: 250, 375, 500 mg Tab: 250, 375, 500 mg Tab SR: 500, 750, 1000 mg Inj: 100, 500 mg/ml	Ventricular and supraventricular arrhythmias, WPW	D: 10-30 mg/kg q 6 h PO (SR q 8 h PO) 5-15 mg/kg q 6 h IM 2 mg/kg IV over 3-5 min up to total dose of 20 mg/kg 20-50 μg/kg/min CRI C: 3-8 mg/kg q 6-8 h IM, PO	Beware hypotension with IV administration Effects increased by high potassium and decreased by low potassium Monitor ECG: 25% prolongation of QRS is sign of toxicity Fewer GI and CV side effects than quinidine Use with caution in cats Reduce dose with severe renal and liver disease

Anti-Arrhythmic Drugs

Drug	Formulation	Indications	Dog Dose (D) Cat Dose (C)	Comments
Propantheline bromide	Tab: 7.5, 15 mg	Sinus bradycardia, AV block, sick sinus syndrome	D: Small: 7.5 mg q 8-12 h Medium: 15 mg PO Large: 30 mg PO C: 7.5 mg q 24 h PO	Sugar coated tablets difficult to halve
Propranolol (Inderal)	Tab: 10, 20, 40, 60, 80, 90 mg Inj: 1 mg/ml Solution: 4, 8, 80 mg/ml	Atrial and ventricular arrhythmias, hypertrophic cardiomyopathy, hypertension, thyrotoxicosis	D: 0.2-1.0 mg/kg q 8 h PO (titrate to effect); 0.02-0.06 mg/kg IV over 5-10 min C: 2.5-10 mg q 8-12 h PO (titrate gradually up to effect) 0.02-0.06 mg/kg IV over 5-10 min	Nonselective β blocker Start with low dose and titrate to effect Taper dose when discontinuing therapy Reduce dose with liver disease
Quinidine gluconate (Quinaglute Dura-tabs)	Tab: 324 mg Inj: 80 mg/ml	Ventricular and supra-ventricular arrhythmias, WPW, conversion of atrial fibrillation	D: 6-20 mg/kg q 6 h PO, IM 6-20 mg/kg q 8 h PO with sustained release products 5-10 mg/kg IV (very slowly) C: None	Decrease digoxin dose 50% when using quinidine Effects increased by high potassium and decreased by low potassium Monitor ECG: 25% prolongation of QRS is sign of toxicity Has vagolytic, negative inotropic and vasodilating properties Hypotension is common with IV administration Reduce dose in CHF, hepatic disease, and hypoalbuminemia
Quinidine polygalac-turonate (Cardioquin)	Tab: 275 mg/ml		Note: Dose calculated for quinidine base equivalent, which varies with each quinidine salt	*Quinidine base (%) in each quinidine salt:* Quinidine sulfate (83%): 200 mg tab = 166 mg quinidine Quinidine gluconate (62%): 324 mg tab = 200 mg quinidine Quinidine polygalacturonate (60%): 275 mg tab = 166 mg quinidine
Quinidine sulfate (Quinidex)	Tab: 100, 200, 300, mg Tab SR: 300 mg Cap: 200, 300 mg Inj:200 mg/ml			

Drug (Brand)	Strength	Indications	Dose	Comments
Sotalol (Betapace)	Tab: 80, 160, 240 mg	Ventricular arrhythmias	D: 1-2 mg/kg q 12 h PO C: None	β blocking (Class 2) effects in addition to Class 3 antiarrhythmic effects Reduce dose with renal disease
Theophylline (Theo-Dur)	Theo-Dur Tab: 100, 200, 300, 450 mg Cap: 50, 75, 125, 200 mg	Asthma, COPD, sinus bradycardia, sick sinus syndrome	D: 9 mg/kg q 8 h PO Theo-Dur: 20 mg/kg q 12 h PO C: 4 mg/kg q 8-12 h PO Theo-Dur: 25 mg/kg q 24 h PO at night	Reduce dose with CHF, liver disease, cimetidine, erythromycin, propranolol Therapeutic range: 10-20 μg/ml Dose on lean body weight
Tocainide (Tonocard)	Tab: 400, 600 mg	Ventricular arrhythmias	D: 10-20 mg/kg q 8 h PO C: None	Oral analog of lidocaine Giving with food may decrease GI upset
Verapamil (Calan, Isoptin)	Tab: 40, 80, 120 mg Inj: 2.5 mg/ml	Supraventricular arrhythmias, hypertrophic cardiomyopathy	D: 0.05-0.2 mg/kg slow IV (1-2 min) in boluses of 0.05 mg/kg given at 10-30 min intervals (to effect) 1-3 mg/kg q 6-8 h PO C: None	Diltiazem is a safer alternative in heart failure Potent vasodilator and negative inotrope

For many of the drugs listed in this formulary, adequate safety and efficacy studies have not been performed in cats and dogs. Doses and indications listed in this formulary were derived from the most current available information at the time of this publication. Adverse effects and precautions listed include only some of those that are possible, or that may have been reported in people. The authors are not responsible for adverse effects or toxicity occurring in patients when drugs are used according to the guidelines used in this formulary. For drugs listed in this formulary, brand names may be listed as examples only. Other brand names may exist and by listing a particular brand name the authors are not advancing one.

Recommended Textbook Readings

1. Allen, D.G., and Kruth, S.A.: *Small Animal Cardiopulmonary Medicine*. Toronto, B.C. Decker, 1988.

2. Bonagura, J.D. (Ed.): *Contemporary Issues in Small Animal Practice; Cardiology*. Volume 7. New York, Churchill Livingstone, 1987.

3. Burtnick, N.L., and Degernes, L.A.: Electrocardiography on fifty-nine anesthetized convalescing raptors. In *Raptor Biomedicine*. Chapter 20. Edited by P.T. Redig, J.D. Remple, and D.B. Hunter. Minneapolis, University of Minnesota Press, 1993.

4. Chung, E.K.: *Manual of Cardiac Arrhythmias*. New York, York Medical Books, 1986.

5. Collet, M., and LeBobinnec, G.: *Electrocardiagraphie et rhythmologie canines*. Paris, Editions du Point Veterinaire, 1991.

6. Detweiter, D.K.: The dog electrocardiogram: A critical review. *In Comprehensive Electrocardiography: Theory and Practice in Health and Disease*. Edited by P.W. MacFarland and T.D.V. Lawrie. New York, Pergamon Press, 1988.

7. Edwards, N.J.: *Bolton's Handbook of Canine and Feline Electrocardiography*. 2nd Edition. Philadelphia, W.B. Saunders, 1987.

8. Ettinger, S.J., and Suter, P.F.: *Canine Cardiology*. Philadelphia, W.B. Saunders, 1970.

9. Fish, C.: *Electrocardiography of Arrhythmias*. Philadelphia, Lea & Febiger, 1990.

10. Fox, P.S. (Ed.): *Canine and Feline Cardiology*. New York, Churchill Livingstone, 1990.

11. Friedman, H.H.: *Diagnostic Electrocardiography and Vectorcardiography*. 3rd Edition. New York, McGraw-Hill, 1985.

12. Gompf, B., Tilley, L.P., and Harpster, N. (Eds.): *Nomenclature and Criteria in Diseases of the Heart and Vessels (Small Animal Medicine)*. Denver, American Animal Hospital Association and The Academy of Veterinary Cardiology, 1986.

13. Hamlin, R.L. (Guest Ed.): *Efficacy of cardiac therapy*. Vet. Clin. North Am. (Small Anim. Pract.), 21(5): 1991.

14. Horwitz, L.N.: *Current Management of Arrhythmias.* Philadelphia, B.C. Decker, 1991.

15. Liu, S-K., Hsu, F.S., and Lee, R.C.T.: *An Atlas of Cardiovascular Pathology.* Taiwan, Wonder Enterprise, 1989.

16. Mandel, W.J.: Cardiac Arrhythmias: *Their Mechanisms, Diagnosis, and Management.* Philadelphia, J.B. Lippincott, 1987.

17. Marriott, H.J.L., and Conover, M.B.: *Advanced Concepts in Arrhythmias.* 2nd Edition. St. Louis, C.V. Mosby, 1989.

18. Miller, M.S., Tilley, L.P., and Detweiler, D.K.: *Cardiac electrophysiology. In Duke's Physiology.* 11th Edition. Edited by M.J. Swenson. Ithaca, N.Y., Cornell University, 1993.

19. Murtaugh, R.J, and Kaplan, P.M.: *Veterinary Emergency and Critical Care Medicine.* St. Louis, Mosby Yearbook, 1991.

20. Pick, A., and Langendorf, R.: *Interpretation of Complex Arrhythmias.* Philadelphia, Lea & Febiger, 1979.

21. Tilley, L.P., Miller, M.S., and Smith, F.W.K.: *Canine and Feline Cardiac Arrhythmias-Self Assessment*, Philadelphia, Lea & Febiger, 1993.

22. Tilley, L.P. (Guest Ed.): *Cardiopulmonary diagnostic techniques.* Vet. Clin. North Am. (Small Anim. Pract.) 13(2): 1983.

23. Tilley, L.P.: *Essentials of Canine and Feline Electrocardiography. Interpretation and Treatment.* 3rd Edition. Philadelphia, Lea & Febiger, 1992.

24. Tilley, L.P. (Guest Ed.): *Feline cardiology.* Vet. Clin. North Am. (Small Anim. Pract.), 7(2): 1977.

25. Tilley, L.P., and Owens, J.M.: *Manual of Small Animal Cardiology.* New York, Churchill Livingstone, 1985.

26. Tilley, L.P., Smith, F.W.K., and Miller, M.S.: *Cardiology Pocket Reference.* 2nd Edition. Denver, American Animal Hospital Association, 1993.

27. Tilley, L.P., and Smith, F.W.K., (Eds.): Diagnostics-Electrocardiography. In *The 5 Minute Veterinary Consult.* Baltimore, Williams & Wilkins, 1997.

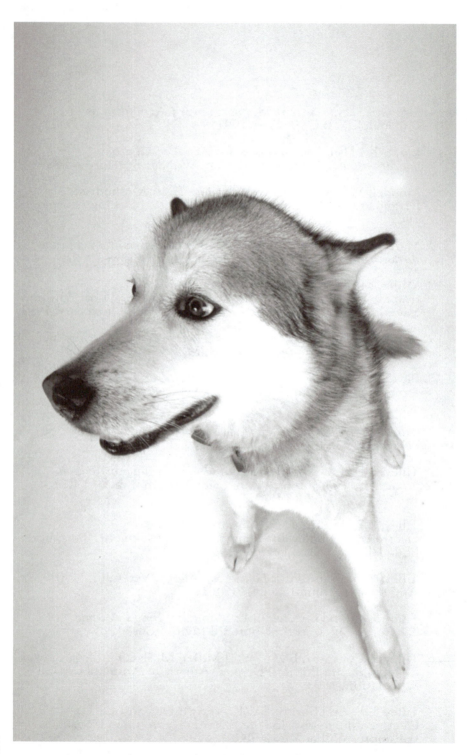